Tai Chi Push Hands

DAVID GRANTHAM
DR. YANG, JWING-MING

Tai Chi Push Hands
THE MARTIAL FOUNDATION OF TAI CHI CHUAN

YMAA Publication Center, Inc.
Wolfeboro, NH USA

YMAA Publication Center, Inc.
PO Box 480
Wolfeboro, NH 03894
800 669-8892 • www.ymaa.com • info@ymaa.com

ISBN: 9781594396458 (print) • ISBN: 9781594396465 (ebook)

This book set in Adobe Garamond and Trade Gothic.

Copyright © 2020 by David Grantham and Dr. Yang, Jwing-Ming
Cover design by Axie Breen
Photos by YMAA Publication Center unless otherwise noted.
Illustration enhancements by Quentin Lopes

20201101

Publisher's Cataloging in Publication

Names: Yang, Jwing-Ming, 1946- author. | Grantham, David W., 1965- author.

Title: Tai chi push hands : the martial foundation of tai chi chuan / Dr. Yang, Jwing-Ming and David Grantham.

Other titles: Title.

Description: Wolfeboro, NH USA : YMAA Publication Center, Inc., [2020] | Series: True wellness. | Includes translation and glossary of Chinese terms. | Includes bibliographical references and index.

Identifiers: ISBN: 9781594396458 (print) | 9781594396465 (ebook) | LCCN: 2020943116

Subjects: LCSH: Tai chi. | Martial arts--Training. | Hand-to-hand fighting, Oriental--Training. | Qi gong. | Qi (Chinese philosophy) | Laozi. Dao de jing. | Force and energy. | Vital force. | Martial arts--Health aspects. | Mind and body. | BISAC: HEALTH & FITNESS / Tai Chi. | HEALTH & FITNESS / Exercise / Stretching. | SPORTS & RECREATION / Martial Arts. | SPORTS & RECREATION / Health & Safety.

Classification: LCC: GV504 .Y366 2020 | DDC: 796.815/5--dc23

Printed in Canada.

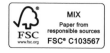

Editorial Notes

Romanization of Chinese Words

The interior of this book primarily uses the Pinyin romanization system of Chinese to English. In some instances, a more popular word may be used as an aid for reader convenience, such as "tai chi" in place of the Pinyin spelling, taiji. Pinyin is standard in the People's Republic of China and in several world organizations, including the United Nations. Pinyin, which was introduced in China in the 1950s, replaces the older Wade-Giles and Yale systems.

Some common conversions are found in the following:

Pinyin	Also spelled as	Pronunciation
qi	chi	chē
qigong	chi kung	chē gōng
qin na	chin na	chǐn nǎ
gongfu	kung fu	gōng foo
taijiquan	tai chi chuan	tī jē chǔén

For more information, please refer to *The People's Republic of China: Administrative Atlas*, *The Reform of the Chinese Written Language*, or a contemporary manual of style.

Formats and Treatment of Chinese Words

Transliterations are provided frequently: for example, *Five Animal Sport* (*Wu Qin Xi*, 五禽戲)

Chinese persons' names are presented mostly in their more popular English spelling. Capitalization is according to the *Chicago Manual of Style* 16th edition. The author or publisher may use a specific spelling or capitalization in respect to the living or deceased person. For example, Cheng, Man-ch'ing can be written as Zheng Manqing.

Photographs

Many photographs include motion arrows to help show the starting position of the body motion.

Dedication

The authors would like to dedicate this book to Dr. Yang's first taijiquan teacher, grandmaster Kao, Tao (高濤). Without grandmaster Kao's teaching, Dr. Yang and his students would not have the firm foundation in taijiquan theory and practice they have today.

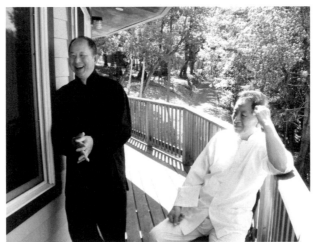

Photo by Jonathan Chang

Table of Contents

Foreword

Dr. Yang Jwing-Ming has been a person of great consequence in the world of Chinese martial arts for some decades. In order to pass on his considerable knowledge and skills, he established original schools in the U.S. and in other countries, and later he founded a classic mountain retreat center, and those unique institutions have provided platforms for matchless in-person teaching. His extensive writings and videos have reached practitioners world-wide who otherwise would not have any opportunity for study with this masterful instructor. I am one of countless practitioners and teachers whose paths have been well influenced by our interactions with Dr. Yang and by his publications.

Mr. Grantham again brings his training and experiences to this latest publication within the continuing body of YMAA materials. One looks forward to more from him in the future.

Teachers of pushing hands recognize that one of the most challenging tasks in giving directions is to find the right words not only to help students realize what it is that they need to do, but also to explain the reasons why it needs to be part of their studies. When such instruction is conveyed in the form of written words rather than in live interaction, it is even more essential that the information should be perfectly stated, clear, and well-ordered. Dr. Yang and Mr. Grantham have collaborated successfully to meet those requirements.

This book will be a useful resource to taijiquan players at all levels of pushing hands experience. It is a welcome reference for teachers looking for solid material. And it can be an inspiration to practitioners who aspire to excellence in taijiquan and who wish for a kind of manual that has accessible and usable information on what to do and how to do it.

Pat Rice
Director, A Taste of China (retired)
Director, Shenandoah Taijiquan Center and Shenandoah Wushu
Director, Winchester Center of the International Yang Family Tai Chi Association
Winchester, Virginia, USA
August 2020

Foreword

To move continuously without breaking is a characteristic of taijiquan. Even when outwardly visible movement pauses, intention continues and unifies the practice. Over the hundreds of years of taijiquan history, one can see the ebb and flow of the art itself through the literary contributions of masters and enthusiasts. Especially during the era of the internet, an abundance of publications, videos, blogs, and discussion groups provide a flood of information. Some repeat the lessons of earlier generations, others postulate new theories. We truly stand on the shoulders of giants and must respect tradition as we make progress. Following the rule of yin and yang, we absorb existing information, adhere to the principles, and bring forth our ideas. These are also the skills of push hands, the embodiment of the taijiquan theories.

Mr. David Grantham and Dr. Yang Jwing-Ming have written a new book on taiji push hands, which presents a great deal of valuable information for practitioners of all levels. Published in a time of pandemic quarantine when the partner work vital to the study of taijiquan is largely unavailable, this book provides a chance to deeply explore these skills in preparation for partner training. As in their 2010 work Tai Chi Ball Qigong, this new offering provides the perspectives of two generations. Both books keep the traditions relevant and fresh while serving as models for the next generations.

It is my honor and pleasure to write this foreword. I wish the authors continued success, and I look forward to their next endeavor!

Nick Gracenin
DC Tai Chi
Washington, DC
August 2020

Preface

For many years, taijiquan has been recognized as an effective method of training the mind and body for a healthy lifestyle. Countless studies demonstrate the various benefits of practicing taijiquan: balance, lowering blood pressure, strengthening of heart and muscle tissue, relieving stress, increasing concentration, and even possibly reversing the signs of aging. It is clear why the popularity of taijiquan has increased.

However, this is only one part of the full benefit of taijiquan. The deeper meaning of taijiquan is in the benefits of the yang side of the training, the fighting art. This book provides the means to begin a quest into seeking this side of the art. We provide theory and exercises to increase the awareness of the mind and body for pushing hands. Keep in mind that there are many styles of taijiquan training and this book can only offer the knowledge and training the authors have experienced through Yang-style taijiquan. Nevertheless, we think that this book along with the many taijiquan DVDs available at YMAA Publication Center, in addition to attending various pushing hands seminars, will assist you in your exploration of many unanswered questions. Our vision is that this information will be used to increase the skill level of the Yang side of taijiquan. With this knowledge, taijiquan will once again prosper and grow further in popularity.

David Grantham

Preface

Taijiquan practice has become very popular since 1960 around the world. Taijiquan not only brings a practitioner a peaceful and relaxed mind and body but can also enhance the body's qi circulation. Qi's circulation has been well known in Chinese medicine as a crucial key to health and longevity. It has been proven that taijiquan practice is able to ease blood pressure, heal some level of arthritis, help elders improve their balance, and treat many forms of spinal illness.

However, due to the emphasis on the health benefits of taijiquan practice, the most important essence of taijiquan, the martial foundation, has been widely ignored. Though taijiquan practice has become popular, it also has become shallow. Taijiquan was created based on the martial applications, which were used for self-defense. Every movement of taijiquan has its unique martial purpose. Without this martial root, taijiquan practice will be just like a form of dancing, without deep meaning and feeling.

Traditionally, after taijiquan practitioners completed learning the taijiquan sequence, they would step into pushing hands practice. From pushing hands practice, a practitioner will be able to sense and exchange qi and feeling with a partner. This is a crucial key and bridge to lead a taijiquan beginner into the path of application and defense training.

In this book, with co-author Mr. David Grantham, we introduce this pushing hands art to those who are interested in pursuing a deeper understanding of and feeling for taijiquan practice. I hope this book and related DVDs will encourage taijiquan practitioners to search for deeper aspects of taijiquan practice.

Dr. Yang, Jwing-Ming 楊俊敏博士
YMAA CA Retreat Center

How to Use This Book

There are so many people practicing taijiquan in the world today; however, very few of them really comprehend the meaning of taijiquan. Taijiquan is a martial art style developed in a Chinese Daoist monastery located in Wudang Mountain (武當山), Hubei Province (湖北省) during the Song Dynasty (AD 960–1279) (宋朝). The monks developed this martial system for the following important purposes:

1. To develop a high level of self-discipline through martial arts training. It requires much self-discipline to reach a high level of martial skills. Monks needed this self-discipline to develop and cultivate their spirit to a higher level to understand the meaning of life. It has been understood that spiritual evolution can be achieved only by conquering the self. Without this conquest, spiritual development will be shallow.

2. To reach spiritual enlightenment. One of the main goals for Daoist spiritual cultivation is to reopen the third eye to reach enlightenment. Martial arts training provided the tools required to reach this goal. This is because in order to reach a high level of martial arts skills, you need a high level of mental focus and qi cultivation. These two elements are the crucial keys to reopen the third eye.

3. To attain health and longevity. The side benefit of the mental and physical training of martial arts is a healthy and long life. When monks lived in remote mountain areas, the emotional disturbances were fewer, the air and the water were fresh, and the lifestyle was simpler. Under this healthy environment, the monks were able to train and to develop a peaceful, calm, and relaxed mind and body.

4. To develop self-defense capabilities. The capability of self-defense was important when monks traveled from one place to another because there were so many bandits around the country.

Today, the main purposes of most taijiquan practitioners are:

1. For relaxation and peaceful mind. This is especially important in today's chaotic society. In the modern world, very few people have a peaceful and relaxed mind. Taijiquan provides a way to reach this goal.

2. For health and longevity. Many people practice taijiquan today simply because it is able to heal many diseases such as high blood pressure, asthma, spinal problems, arthritis, and breathing difficulties. Many others practice taijiquan because they are able to prevent sickness and it offers them a chance for a longer, happier life.

Unfortunately, taijiquan as a means to spiritual enlightenment and martial defensive capability has been widely ignored in today's practice. This implies that the level of taijiquan training has also become shallow. Worst of all, the art has lost its original root and essence.

In order to reach to a high level of feeling and spiritual cultivation, we need to trace back taijiquan's root and essence, its martial training, discipline, and meaning. Without these, the forms practiced are just like a routine of relaxed dancing. If that is all it is allowed to be, then those interested in relaxation may just create a relaxed dancing pattern for themselves. There is no need for a teacher.

However, if you wish to feel and understand the meaning of each traditional movement, then you need a qualified and experienced teacher. After all, to reach a high level of martial defense capability, a teacher must know the theory and have good skills of taijiquan fighting capability. Furthermore, they will also need many years of experience through teaching and practice. A qualified teacher is a crucial key for entering the profound depth of this art.

The information in this book is for those who wish to deepen their taijiquan skills. It is a guide for you to train pushing hands and enhance your knowledge of pushing hands theory. Most of the exercises in this book are also found on the various taijiquan DVDs available at YMAA Publication Center (www.ymaa.com). DVD references are noted in the text as appropriate. Keep in mind that not all exercises are found in the DVDs, and some exercises have changed, or evolved, from the time the DVDs were made. As such, it is important to find an instructor or participate in seminars to help you understand how and why these exercises have evolved.

You will also find various references to the theories behind many of the exercises throughout the book. We cannot emphasize enough the importance of studying the theories of taiji pushing hands. Many of the exercises were created by masters who spent countless hours pondering their taijiquan training. This knowledge will help you understand the reasons behind the exercises and provide you with a deeper sense of taijiquan itself. Once you are ready to practice the exercises, begin with the foundational movements of training. As with all martial training, you must develop these fundamental skills before moving on to the two-person skill set. These basic exercises will help develop the mind and body in preparation for encountering your opponent. Do not take these exercises lightly and do not skip them. Proper fundamental training protects against injury and provides the foundation for deeper training. Too many people attempt to rush training and as a result find they were not properly prepared for the next step.

Once you have trained the basics, you will need to have various partners to further train the two-person exercises. It is always a good idea to train with as many people as possible. Training with people of different heights, length of limbs, and varied reactions will enhance your skills. Once again, do not rush the exercises; this is your time to train and enhance your skills. Throughout this phase, you will see the difference in body movements, breathing, mental intent, and qi flow. Your spirit will be lifted. Strength will be less of a factor as sense of awareness increases.

As you pass through the various exercises you may find it necessary to go back to previous exercises and theories to further your knowledge, and we recommend you do so. Finally, realize the information in this book is only one tool for you to train your skills. It is solely based upon the knowledge and experience the authors have gained through their years of training. There are endless amounts of other training tools out there to explore. It is up to you how far and deep you wish to train, and only you can decide which information is important to your life and how hard you will train to achieve your goals.

Chapter 1: Theory of Taiji Pushing Hands

1.1 Introduction

Taiji pushing hands theory is deep and wide and covers many related subjects. With this in mind, it is assumed that you already have a full understanding of certain concepts such as the differences in the definition of taiji and taijiquan. You should also have full understanding of the Thirteen Postures of taijiquan as well as the training theories of qigong. The basic concept of taiji pushing hands is to master the skills of eight basic jing patterns and the Five Steppings (ba men wu bu, 八門五步). Once you have learned and mastered these skills, you will be able to perform pushing hands actions effectively and eventually you will be able to develop your skills of freestyle sparring. Taijiquan practitioners without the knowledge or training in these basic concepts will have lost the taijiquan training essence and their training will remain shallow. It is similar to building a house without first creating a strong foundation. Without a proper base anything built on top of it will eventually crumble. With this in mind, we highly recommend you refer to the various books related to taijiquan at YMAA Publication Center before beginning your pushing hands training.

In the following sections we will first discuss the basic theories of taijiquan pushing hands training. We will then briefly highlight a few basics of rooting and centering. These simple concepts are necessary for becoming proficient in taijiquan pushing hands but are often overlooked. Next we will explore the relationships between yin-yang and taijiquan pushing hands. One should also be aware of substantial and insubstantial actions in taijiquan pushing hands training. Finally, a practitioner must also understand the six turning secrets. These six key training secrets will provide the practitioner with the knowledge of how to transfer their energy back and forth between yin and yang. It is important to know these methods of exchanging so you can comfortably change the movements involved in your interaction and gain control of your opponent.

1.2 About Pushing Hands

When discussing the concept of pushing hands we often envision two individuals engaging in an exercise where one is attempting to find the other's center of gravity (i.e., physical center) and push them off balance. In some cases, the tendencies of aggressive behavior evolve into a competitive interaction between the two individuals, and unfortunately the essence of taiji pushing hands becomes lost, with one person winning the match through use of force. Pushing hands practice involves the application of taijiquan theory and basic movements into matching actions with a partner. To further understand the nature of taiji pushing hands we will explore a few theories written by taijiquan masters.

> Taijiquan uses pushing hands training to practice the applications. Learning pushing hands means learning feeling jing. When there is feeling jing, then understanding jing is not difficult. Therefore, *The Total Thesis (of Taijiquan)* said: "from understanding jing then gradually reach the spiritual enlightenment." There is no doubt that this sentence is rooted in (built upon) pushing hands. Peng (i.e., wardoff), lü (i.e., rollback), ji (i.e., press), and an (i.e., push), four (jing) patterns are the stationary pushing hands of adhering, connecting, attaching, and following which give up self and follow the opponent.[1]
>
> 太極拳以練習推手為致用，學推手則即是學覺勁，有覺勁則懂勁便不難矣。故總論所謂由懂勁而階及神明，此言即根於推手無疑矣。掤、攦、擠、按四式即黏、連、貼、隨舍己從人之定步推手。

Master Yang, Cheng-Fu (楊澄甫) illustrates here that the progression of understanding taijiquan applications is through pushing hands training. Through it you are able to build your skills of feeling. You will also note the emphasis on giving up oneself and following the opponent. By doing so, you will learn to understand your opponent's intention and lead them into emptiness. These four basic jing (勁) patterns of stationary pushing hands are the main essence of learning this.

> To give up myself and follow the opponent is to abandon my idea and follow the opponent's movements. This is the most difficult thing (i.e., training) in taijiquan. Because when two persons are exchanging hands (i.e., combating), the conception of winning and losing is serious. (In this case) the opponent and I will not endure each other, not even mentioning that when mutually (we) are attacking each other or mutually stalemating with each other and (you) are asked to give up your right (of trying to win in a resisting competition). What is called to give up yourself and follow the opponent is not only explained from the words. In our Dao (i.e., the Dao of taijiquan), its hidden meaning is extremely

profound. (In order to understand them and apply them in action) the practitioner must put a gongfu in the four words: solely focus on cultivating the human nature.[2]

捨己從人，是捨棄自己的主張，而依從他人動作。在太極拳中，為最難能之事。因兩人在交手之時，勝負之觀念重，彼我決不相容，何況互相攻擊，或在相持之中，而棄其權利。所謂捨己從人，不僅作字面解釋而矣。在吾道中，其寓意至深。學者當於惟務養性，四字下功夫。

"Four words" means wardoff, rollback, press, and push. From this Wu-style taijiquan secret, we can see that the most profound and difficult part of taiji pushing hands is to release the ego and learn to be aware of incoming forces. We tend to be competitive in nature and at times we allow the emotional bond of the ego and the need to win to control our actions, leading to mutual resistance in a pushing hands engagement. When you are able to let go of your emotion and be patient, you can then allow yourself to follow and adhere to your opponent's will. By learning to cultivate your emotional mind you will learn to manipulate your opponent's intent and lead them to emptiness.

[Leading]: "(When) lead (the coming force) to enter the emptiness, unite and then immediately emit," "(Use) four ounces to repel one thousand pounds." Unification means repelling. If (one) can comprehend this word, (then) he is the one born to wisdom.[3]

《引》：〝引進落空合即出〞，〝四兩撥千斤〞，合即撥也，此字能悟，真夙慧者也。

Master Wǔ, Cheng-Qing (武澄清) further expands upon the concept of leading your opponent into emptiness. Four ounces to repel one thousand pounds is a term common to taijiquan practices and pushing hands training. This basic concept relates to the necessity of using the skills of listening, adhering, and following rather than resisting when engaging your opponent. This process of leading involves the development of unification between you and your opponent's mental intent. Once you understand this you will further understand the depths of taiji pushing hands.

The classic says: "Although in techniques, there are many side doors (i.e., other martial arts styles), after all, it is nothing more than the strong beating the weak." Also says: "Investigate (consider) the saying of four ounces repel one thousand pounds. It is apparent that this cannot be accomplished by strength." That the strong beating the weak is due to the pre-birth natural capability that is born with it. It (the capability) is not obtained through learning. What is called "using the four ounces to repel one thousand pounds" is actually matching the theory of using the balance (i.e., leverage). It does not matter the lightness or the heaviness of the body, the large or the small of the force, can shift the opponent's weighting center, and (finally) move his entire body. Therefore, the reason that the movements of taijiquan are different from other (martial) techniques is because they do not defeat the opponent with force. Furthermore, (it) can not only strengthen the tendons, keep the bones healthy, and harmonize the qi and blood, but also be used to cultivate (i.e., harmonize) the body and (mental) mind, keep away from sickness and extend the life. (It) is a marvelous Dao of post-heaven body cultivation.[4]

經云：〝斯技旁門甚多，概不外有力打無力。〞又曰：〝查四兩撥千斤之句，顯非力勝。〞夫有力打無力，斯乃先天自然之能，生而知之。非學而後能之。所謂四兩撥千斤者，實則合乎權衡之理。無論體之輕重，力之大小，能在動之間，移其重心，使之全身牽動。故太極拳之動作，所以異於他技者，非務以力勝人也。推而進之，不惟強筋健骨，調和氣血，而自能修養身心，卻病延年，為後天養身之妙道焉。

Once again the author reminds us that taijiquan is an art that emphasizes softness in actions. It is different in that it doesn't rely on the stiffness of blocking but instead focuses on matching your opponent through the use of listening and following. The whole body and mind are relaxed and centered. Using this leverage, the individual can move the opponent completely without force.

Ancient people said: "If (one is) able to lead (the coming force) into emptiness, (one) can (use) the four ounces to repel one thousand pounds; if (one is) unable to lead (the coming force) into the emptiness, (one) is unable to (use) the four ounces to repel one thousand pounds." This saying is quite correct and conclusive. The beginners are unable to comprehend (this saying). I would like to add a few sentences to explain this. (This will) allow those practitioners who have strong will to learn these techniques (i.e., taijiquan) and be able to follow the opponent and have progress daily.[5]

昔人云，能引進落空，能四兩撥千斤；不能引進落空，不能四兩撥千斤。語甚賅括。初學末由領悟，予加數語以解之；俾有志斯技者，得以從人，庶日進有功矣。

Master Li, Yi-She (李亦畬) also says that one should understand the concept of using four ounces to repel one thousand pounds of force. Once again, the foundation of taijiquan pushing hands is to lead an incoming force into emptiness. This is done through the skills of listening and following. He goes on to say that the skills of listening and following are necessary for knowing your opponent, which means discerning his intentions and capabilities. Listening and following are also needed to know yourself, which means knowing how to harmoniously coordinate your mind, body, and spirit. You will find the above selection in the book, *Tai Chi Secrets of the Wŭ and Li Styles*, by Dr. Yang, Jwing-Ming available at YMAA Publication Center.

1.3 Taiji Pushing Hands Training Contents

Taiji pushing hands is commonly called "communication" or "question and answer" (wen da, 問答) in taijiquan practice. When you begin taiji pushing hands practice, you are exchanging your mental intent, skills, and qi with your opponent. You are applying your yin and yang sides of taijiquan training into actions with a partner. As such, the feeling (or "listening" in taijiquan) is extremely important. First you must have listening, and then you are able to understand. From understanding, you are able to attach, stick, follow, and connect. These are the crucial keys of taijiquan techniques. In fact, it is from these basic keys that the taijiquan martial skills can be applied.

From these basic practices, you learn how to master the fundamental structure of taijiquan: Thirteen Postures (十三勢). If you are not familiar with these postures and cannot apply them in action, your taijiquan will have lost its essence and should not be called taijiquan.

The contents of taiji pushing hands can be listed as:

1. Taiji Qigong: learn how to use the mind to lead the qi for action.

2. Balance and Rooting: learn how to keep yourself at the centered, balanced, and rooted position both when stationary and when stepping.

3. Stationary Single Pushing Hands: the first step to teach a beginner how to listen, yield, follow, lead, and neutralize. From single pushing hands, you build a firm foundation of double pushing hands.

4. Stationary Double Pushing Hands: also called "peng, lü, ji, an" (掤、攦、擠、按). A drill teaches you how to use both hands to apply the first four basic structures of taijiquan. The four basic structures are wardoff (peng, 掤), rollback (lü, 攦), press (ji, 擠), and push (an, 按).

5. Moving Single Pushing Hands: learn how to step while applying the basic four postures.

6. Moving Double Pushing Hands: learn how to step while using both hands to apply the basic four postures.

7. Rollback and Press: also commonly called "cai, lie, zhou, kao" (採、挒、肘、靠) and means pluck, split, elbow, and bump. Rollback includes small rollback (xiao lü, 小攦) and large rollback (da lü, 大攦). This practice focuses on mastering the second four of the taijiquan Thirteen Postures.

8. Freestyle Pushing Hands. Once you are able to apply the eight basic jing patterns with smooth and skillful coordination with stepping, then you progress to freestyle pushing hands. Freestyle practice provides a firm foundation for sparring and setups for kicking, striking, wrestling, and qin na.

From the fundamental practice of single pushing hands, advancing into double pushing hands, (you learn) to listen, understand, advance forward, retreat backward, beware of the left, and look to the right. When (you) have reached a natural reactive stage of using the yi without the yi, then (you) may enter the practice of moving pushing hands. (However, you should know that) in moving pushing hands training, the practice of advance forward, retreat backward, beware of the left, look to the right, and central equilibrium also start from single pushing hands. Its main goal is to train central equilibrium so it can harmonize the criteria of advance forward, retreat backward, beware of the left, look to the right. After the hands, the eyes, the body movements, the techniques, and the stepping can be coordinated and harmonized with each other, then (you can) enter the practice of double pushing hands, large rollback, and small rollback of stepping moving pushing hands. Afterward, (you can) enter the practice of taijiquan sparring. From the practice of sparring, (you) should continue to search deeper for profound understanding, experience, and applications. After a long period of practice, the moving of the Five Steppings can be carried out as you wish.

由定步單推手晉為雙推手之基本練習中，而聽、而懂，而進、而退、而顧、而盼。在達乎意不為意之自然反應後，即能步入動步推手練習。動步之進、退、顧、盼、與中定亦由單推手始。其主要目的在訓練行步中之中定與步伐之進、退、顧、盼也。在手、眼、身、法、步能合諧調配得宜後，即步入雙推手與大、小攦之動步練習。之後，即可步入太極散手之練習。在由散手對練中去尋求更深之瞭解、經驗、與應用。久而久之，五步之行隨心所欲也。

After you have mastered all of the basic skills for your body's strategic actions and are familiar with the techniques of applying the eight basic jing patterns in stationary pushing hands, start your pushing hands training while moving. Without mastering these basic skills in the stationary position your body will be tense and stiff while moving. You will be unable to maintain your central equilibrium, your root will be shallow, and your techniques will not be effective. In order to build yourself to a high level of skill, bad habits must be corrected first and basic skills must be reinforced.

When you advance to moving pushing hands, again you must start from moving single pushing hands before progressing to moving double pushing hands. In this stage of training you learn how to maintain your central equilibrium while you are stepping and turning. After you have reached a comfortable level where the yi (mind) does not have to be there (i.e. natural reaction), then you can proceed to large and small rollback (da lü, xiao lü, 大攦、小攦) training. Gradually, you proceed into sparring and other advanced jing skills such as spiraling, coiling, controlling, and borrowing.

The chart of general contents outlines the basic structure and procedures needed to lead a beginner to a proficient level of taijiquan applications. Other than these basic routines, there are many other practices such as:

1. Centering (zhong ding, 中定): basic practice with a partner to develop listening, understanding, yielding, following, leading, and neutralizing. This practice trains the body's central equilibrium.

2. Stationary and Moving Rooting and Balance (zha gen, 紮根): basic training to develop the feeling of your root and to grow it deeper, with a good body balance. It also trains the body's central equilibrium. This training also teaches you how to step with the last five actions of taijiquan the Thirteen Postures: forward, backward, left, right, and central equilibrium.

3. Sense of Distance (ju gan, 距感): training to keep an advantageous distance between you and your opponent. This training further develops your skills of how to step with the last five actions of the taijiquan Thirteen Postures: forward, backward, left, right, and central equilibrium.

4. Angling (she jiao, 設角): training how to occupy empty doors (qiang zhong men, 搶中門) (qiang kong men, 搶空門) and attach from open windows (tian chuang, di hu, 天窗、地戶). This training further develops your skills of how to step with the last five actions of the taijiquan Thirteen Postures: forward, backward, left, right, and central equilibrium.

5. Taiji Fighting Set (san shou dui lian, 散手對練): trains a skillful pushing hands practitioner how to apply the techniques into real sparring.

6. Taiji Sparring (dui da/san da, 對打／散打): this is the final stage of pushing hands.

In addition to the basic routines for training, you should also practice two of the most important and crucial trainings of taijiquan: taiji ball qigong and also yin-yang symbol

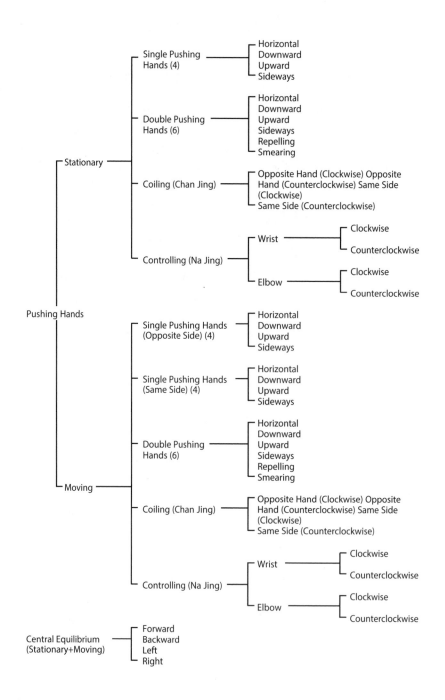

General Contents of Pushing Hands Practice

sticking hands training to improve your pushing hands skills. These two training techniques are discussed later in this book.

Once you have reached this level, you will have accomplished about 50 percent of taijiquan training. Then you gradually include other jings into free sparring such as borrowing jing, jumping jing, and kicking jing.

In the next section, we will summarize the basic structure of taiji pushing hands through rooting and centering.

1.4 Rooting, Uprooting, and Centering

1.4.1 Rooting and Uprooting (zha gen yu ba gen, 紮根與拔根)

Taijiquan is a short and middle range fighting style. In pushing hands situations, both you and your opponent are seeking to find each other's center. Once the center is discovered the next move is to uproot the other person, thus winning the engagement. Keep in mind this occurs simultaneously with respect to finding the center and root. It is important to focus on finding your opponent's center; however, you must also be aware of your own center and rooting, otherwise you will be uprooted or wrestled down to the ground easily by your opponent. In the following section we will highlight a few theories associated with the importance of rooting and centering. If you are interested in seeking further information on this subject it is highly recommended you seek this information out by referring to the taijiquan theory books for further studies.

Taijiquan Classic said: "The root is at the feet, (jing or movement is) generated from the legs, mastered (i.e. controlled) by the waist, and manifested (i.e. expressed) from the fingers. From the feet to the legs to the waist must be integrated, into one unified qi. When moving forward or backward, (you can) then catch the opportunity and gain the superior position. If (you) fail to catch the opportunity and gain the superior position, (your) body will be disordered. To solve this problem, (you) must look to the waist and legs. Up and down, forward and backward, left and right, it's all the same. All of this is done with the yi (mind), not externally." This has clearly implied that the rooting is the most important (point) in taijiquan's offense and defense. When the root is firmed, the central equilibrium will be steady and the jing can be emitted (effectively). If the root is floating, then the central equilibrium will be damaged, the mind will be scattered, and this can be taken advantage of by an opponent.

太極拳經謂："其根在腳，發於腿，主宰於腰，形於手指。由腳而腿而腰，總須完整一氣。向前退後，乃能得機得勢。有不得機得勢處，身便散亂。其病必於腰腿求之。上下前後左右皆然。凡此皆是意，不在外面。"此即意紮根乃太極拳攻防之首要。根穩,中定定,而勁能發。根浮,則中定損,意亂,為敵所乘,置我於不得機之境地。

From this statement of the *Taijiquan Classic* we are reminded of the importance of the root in both taijiquan and pushing hands training. This is where the power initiates ("The root is at the feet. . .") and to disrupt this area will disrupt any intent to control engagement. Firming the root is not a purely external action; it also involves the mind (internal). Without maintaining this balance your mind will be scattered and the body will follow, allowing your opponent to take advantage of the situation and win the battle. If you find yourself losing this balance, you must look to your waist, legs, and feet to re-establish your rooting for defense and jing manifestation.

The most important thing in the training of firming the root is that all the joints must be threaded together and function as a single qi (i.e., single unit). In order to thread the joint together, (you) must first know how to keep the joints light and agile. According to theory, the entire body can be divided into upper, middle, and lower sections. From the knees and below is the lower section, from the knees to xinkan (i.e. jiuwei) is the middle section, and from xinkan to the neck and head is the upper section. When the root of the lower section is firmed, the middle section can be relaxed, and the jing manifested from the upper level can be strong. To reach the steadiness and firmness of the root in the lower section, (you) must begin (your training) from ankles, knees, and hips, these three joint places. If these three places can be loosened, soft, agile, and alive, then the root can be firmed. However, the most important of all is to keep the waist area soft. When the waist is soft, you can control the jing, and emitting or neutralizing can be swift and natural. In that case, it will be hard for (your) opponent's jing to reach your center and pull your root.

紮根之首要,在於節節貫穿,全身完整一氣。為求貫穿,必先懂得關節之輕靈。依理而言,全身可分為上、中、下三盤。由膝而下為之下盤,由膝至心坎為中盤,由心坎至頭頂為上盤。下盤跟穩,中盤能鬆,上盤之勁顯必強。為求下盤之根穩,必先由踝、膝、胯三處關節著手。若此三關節能鬆,能軟,能靈,能活,則根可定。然最重者,乃是鬆腰。腰鬆則勁可為我主宰,發、化靈活自然。如此,敵之勁必難達於我之中心,並拔其根。

The entire body is connected by joints. Through these joints, your opponent's power can reach your root and destroy it. In taijiquan, the body acts as a single soft whipping unit. Jing is initiated from the root, controlled by the waist, and manifested in the fingers.

In order to make this happen, the joints must be soft, relaxed (i.e., light), and activated. These conditions are required not just for the jing's manifestation, but also to prevent the opponent's power from reaching your root.

The body can be divided into three sections (san pan, 三盤): from the knees down, from the knees to xinkan (心坎) (jiuwei, Co-15) (鳩尾), and from xinkan to the crown. Xinkan is a martial arts term for the cavity named jiuwei in Chinese medicine. Xinkan is the lower part of the sternum. In Chinese martial arts training, the lower section (from the knees down) is considered the most important since it is related to your root and stability. If you do not have a firm root and good stability, your mind and physical body will float, and your concentration and spirit will be shallow. In this case, your power cannot be manifested effectively, and you will

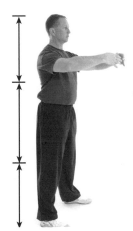

The body's three sections.

have provided your opponent with an advantageous position from which to destroy your center and take you down.

In order to have firm root and stability, you must first have strong legs, especially the joints in the ankles, knees, and hips. You must also be able to control them efficiently so they can be soft and loose as well. You must, in addition, have a waist that can be controlled by your mind efficiently. For all of this, you must also learn precision of control so that when it is necessary to be hard, the joints can be hard, and when they must be soft, they can be soft. When this happens, your mind will be able to govern the middle and the lower section of the body effectively for any defensive or offensive situation.

Generally, the distance between your physical center (i.e., gravity) and the ground registered in your subconscious mind was constantly adjusted as you grew taller. From this subconscious mind, we can pull our root any time and walk. If this distance in our subconscious mind is too long, then the root will be too deep and it will be hard to step. If this distance in our subconscious mind is too short, then the root is floating and you can fall. Normally, in order to increase the level of stability (i.e., rooting) we sink down to lower the physical center. Consequently, the distance between the gravity center and the ground is extended into the ground. Thus, we are rooted.

人體物理中心與地面之距離，一般人之潛意識，隨身體之成長而調節。由此潛意識，吾等可隨時拔根而步行。如此潛意識之距離太長，則根沈而難行。如此潛意識之距離太短，則根浮而易傾。平時，為增加身體之穩度，我們下蹲身勢以降低身體之物理中心，同時潛意識理物理中心與地面之距離，往地裡伸展。由此，根紮矣。

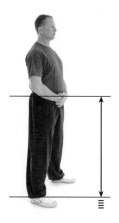

The distance between your physical gravity center and the ground.

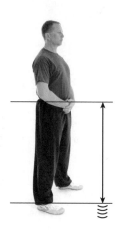

If your mind registers the distance as shorter than the distance from your physical center to the ground, you cannot walk.

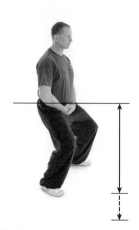

Building a stronger root.

Theoretically, since the day you learned how to walk, your mind has been registering the distance between your physical gravity center and the ground (0033). This distance was adjusted during the course of your growth. It is from the recognition of this distance that you can walk. If the distance in your mind is longer than this distance and sinks into the ground, then you cannot walk. On the contrary, if the distance in your mind is shorter than this distance, then your mind is above the ground and you are not rooted in walking. In this case, you will be floating and awkward. Generally, in order to build a stronger root you squat down to lower your physical center of gravity. Training in a squat builds physical strength and trains your mind to go underneath the ground to establish a firm root.

In Chinese martial arts training, there are two ways of establishing a stronger root; one is through physical stances and the other is through breathing and mental training that allows you to extend the distance from your physical gravity center into the ground. Both kinds of training are required.

Uprooting is used against the opponent, to destroy his root, and to put him at a disadvantage. In order to pull his root, (you) must first destroy his central equilibrium. When the central equilibrium is disrupted, his mind will be disordered and his qi will float. Seize this opportunity and pull his root off. In order to destroy his central equilibrium, (you) must know listening, following, attaching, and adhering jings. Attach to his center and adhere to his skin and muscles. Yin and yang mutually exchange. Capture his central door and occupy his empty door to confuse his mind. In this case, (you) will put (your) opponent into a disadvantageous position that can be used by you to destroy his central equilibrium. When the central equilibrium is destroyed, the root can be easily pulled.

拔根乃我對待敵人，以損其根，並置敵於不利之地。欲拔敵根，必先損其中定。中定損，其意必亂，其氣必浮，趁此良機，拔其根也。欲損其中定，必懂聽、隨、沾、黏之勁。沾其中心，黏其肌膚，陰陽交替，搶其中門，佔其空門，以亂其心。如此，囗必置敵於不利，為我所用並損其中定。中定損，根易拔矣。

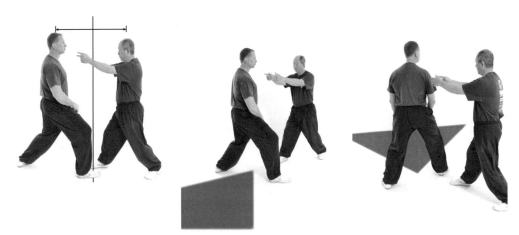

The central door.   The empty door front side.   The empty door rear side.

In order to create an opportunity for your attack, first you must put your opponent into a defensive and urgent situation. One of the most common ways to do this is to destroy his balance and root. When this happens, your opponent must pay attention to his balance and root and try to re-establish it. You will have created an advantageous situation for your attack. However, in order to reach this goal, you must first be good in the skills of listening, understanding, following, attaching, and adhering jings. With the skillfulness and effectiveness of these jings, you will be able to place your opponent into a defensive situation. You must also be an expert in using the exchangeable yin-yang strategies to confuse your opponent. Once you have created these advantageous opportunities, you should then immediately occupy the central door (zhong men, 中門) or reposition yourself and enter his empty door (kong men, 空門). The central door is a shoulder-width area in between two opponents when facing each other. Once you have occupied this position, you will have put your opponent into an urgent situation. Empty door means the door is opened that allows you to step in for an attack. This area is located in front as well as in back of the opponent. Once you have seized this door, your opponent will feel naked and exposed to your attack.

Taijiquan Classic said: "If there is a top, there is a bottom; if there is a front, there is a back; if there is a left, there is a right. If yi (wisdom mind) wants to go upward, this implies considering downward. (This means) if (you) want to lift and defeat an opponent, you must first consider his root. When the opponent's root is broken, he will inevitably be defeated quickly and certainly." This can be done through the application of yin and yang strategies of exchange. When the opponent's mind is disordered, the root can be pulled. In order to pull his root, (you) must first trick him with downward tactics to entice his mind upward. When his mind is upward, you immediately take this opportunity to pull his root. Knowing is easier than actually executing it; therefore, learners should keep practicing until the skills can be carried out effectively.

經云："有上即有下，有前即有後，有左即有右。如意要向上，即寓下意。若將物掀起，而加以挫之之意。斯其根自斷，乃壞之速而無疑。"此即意陰陽交替而用，敵心一亂，根可拔矣。欲拔其根，必先寓下意，以引敵上提之意。敵意一上提，我即趁機拔其根也。知易行難，學者必多習之以為效。

In order to pull the opponent's root, you must know how to use insubstantial (i.e., yin) and substantial (i.e., yang) tactics skillfully. This will confuse your opponent. For example, in order to pull up, you must first pull down. When the opponent resists with upward intention and action, then you follow his action and immediately pull up. In order to make him fall to the left, first you apply pressure to his left (your right). Once he has initiated a reactive action against your force, then you immediately change your force to your left and make him lose balance. Through these on-off and off-on actions, you will put your opponent into a defensive and disorienting position that you control.

1.4.2 Central Equilibrium (Zhong Ding, 中定)

Equally as important in pushing hands training is centering. Centering can also be defined as central equilibrium and is considered the second most important posture of the Thirteen Postures (shi san shi, 十三勢) of taijiquan training. This posture is associated with the earth element and is tied closely to rooting. The following are a few theories written by masters of taijiquan that demonstrate why it is necessary to be aware of your center in push hands training.

> Central equilibrium, advance forward, retreat backward, beware of the left, and look to the right should be practiced in stationary pushing hands. Central equilibrium involves balance, rooting, and making sure "the head is suspended." Advance and retreat involves the upper body's advance and retreat. This advance and retreat can be accomplished from the exchange of the climbing mountain stance (i.e., bow and arrow stance) and four-six stance. Mountain climbing stance is mainly used for advancing, offense, and sealing, while four-six stance is mainly used for retreating, defense, and yielding. Beware of the left and look to the right are carried out from the upper body's turning and mainly used for leading, neutralizing, and controlling.

> 定步中定之勢與定步之進、退、顧、盼由定步推手練起。中定者，平衡、紮根、頂勁之謂也。進、退者，由腰而上身體之進與退也。此進退由蹬山步（弓箭步）與四六步之轉換而成。蹬山步主進、主攻、主封，四六步主退、主守、主讓。顧、盼者，由腰而上身體之輾轉而成，主引、主化、主拿也。

From this statement one sees the importance of training the central equilibrium. Training your central equilibrium involves keeping both the mind and body centered through rooting techniques. Your head should also feel as though it is suspended. This means the crown of the head feels as though it is uplifted toward the sky with the chin slightly tucked inward. In order to reach all of these goals, you must know how to be relaxed and soft. Without these two criteria, your body will be tensed, your mind will be scattered, your root will be shallow, and your listening and understanding jings will be dull.

The author continues to describe the applications of the mountain climbing (deng shan bu, 登山步) (or bow and arrow stance) (gong jian bu, 弓箭步) and four-six stances (si liu bu, 四六步) of taijiquan practice. Again, the importance of central equilibrium plays an important factor here. No matter which direction you choose to move in it should be the whole body moving as one unit. To not maintain this central posture is to lean while moving and will allow you to be defeated easily by causing you to fall off balance.

> Before the action of extending, bending, opening, and closing is called center. Extremely quiet (i.e., calm) without movement is called steady (i.e., equilibrium, balanced, and rooted). The heart (i.e., emotional mind) and the qi are clean and harmonious, the spirit of vitality reaches the top (of the head), no tilting no leaning, is the qi of central equilibrium. It is also the root of the Dao (i.e., taijiquan).[6]
>
> 伸屈開合之未發謂之中。寂然不動謂之定，心氣清和，精神貫頂，不偏不倚，是為中定之氣，亦道之本也。

From this statement we see that if you keep your mind in the center of gravity (i.e., real dan tian, 真丹田) you are in the wuji state. There is no intent; both the physical and mental centers remain in this central state. Your mind is calm and you sink your qi to the lower dan tian to build your root and lead qi up the top of your head to build up your spirit of vitality. Doing so will allow you to have a firm root and high spirit, thus leading you to act with balance. All your movements in taijiquan training build upon having a central equilibrium. Without this feeling you will be tense, allowing your mind to scatter with emotion, and ultimately you will find yourself uprooted.

> Keep the central earth (customary name is standing on the post): When there is steadiness, then there is a root. First understand the four sides of the body's advancing and retreating clearly. Then wardoff (peng), rollback (lü), press (ji), and push (an) four hands (i.e., techniques) can automatically (be) manifested as wished. To gain the truth (of these four techniques), (you) must spend (a great deal) of gongfu. When the body's shape, waist, and crown of the head are all regulated correctly, the yi (i.e., wisdom mind) and the qi in attaching, adhering, connecting, and following will be uniform (i.e., smooth). Correspond (i.e., coordinate) the movements and the feeling mutually, the spirit is the sovereign, and the bones and the meat (i.e., muscles) are the subjects. Clearly discriminate the seventy-two stages of maturity. Naturally, you will gain both martial (i.e., physical) and scholar (i.e., internal cultivation or understanding) capabilities.[7]
>
> 守中土〔俗名站樁〕：定之方中有根，先明四正進退身。掤、攦、擠、按自四手，須費功夫得其真。身形腰頂皆可以 ，粘、黏、連、隨意氣均。運動知覺來相應，神是君位骨肉臣。分明火候七十二，天然乃武並乃文。

The word zhong tu (中土) refers to central earth, or central equilibrium. Here it is referring to the second most important posture of the Thirteen Postures. In order to reach a high level of central equilibrium one begins with fundamental stances such as horse stance (ma bu, 馬步). These stances would often be trained on posts (zhan zhuang, 站樁) to assist in rooting and centering skills by focusing the mind well below the ground. Once you have mastered this you would follow through the Five Steppings then the eight basic jing patterns, thus completing the Thirteen Postures. Throughout the movements the body will be trained to remain upright, the waist will be loose, and the mind centered. Additionally, there must be a clear communication between the body and mind. The physical body will listen to the commands of the mind, and the mind will understand the opponent's intent through feeling of the body. This mutual correspondence will allow you to gain internal (scholar) and external (martial) awareness. You will see the reference to seventy-two stages. This demonstrates the progression of any achievement. Progression is a time-honored art with many levels leading to deep understanding and knowledge.

> In order to keep the central equilibrium of the physical center, steadiness of the qi's entrance and exit, and stability of the xin (i.e., emotional mind) and yi (i.e., wisdom mind). The most important thing is to keep the waist and kua (thighs and hip joints area) loose. The waist is the connecting place of the upper body and the lower body. When the waist is loose, the root can be firm and the top and the bottom can be harmonized with each other. When the waist is loose, the body will naturally be loose. When the body can be loose, then the yi can be concentrated. When the yi can be concentrated, the xin will be peaceful. When the xin is peaceful, then the spirit will have its center. When the spirit has its center, then the body and the mind are all steady.
>
> 為持身體物理中心之定，氣能進出丹田自如之定，心與意之定，其首要在於鬆腰鬆胯也。腰為上身下體關連之所，腰鬆則根穩，上下相合。腰能鬆，則身能鬆，身能鬆，則意專，意專則心安，心安則神有主矣。神有主，則身心均定矣。

To be in a state of central equilibrium a person must be rooted with a relaxed waist and calm mind. In order to keep this area loose and relaxed you must learn to train the waist and joints of the hips (i.e., internal and external kua) (nei kua, wai kua, 內胯、外胯). When this central place is loose and comfortable, the qi can flow in and out easily, and the mind can be sensitive in this place and steady. When these places are loose, you will be able to protect your root. When your root is firmed, the center can be protected. In this case, you can protect your center and keep the equilibrium.

The practicing method for maintaining central equilibrium is to allow your partner to control your elbows and find your center. His intention is to destroy your central equilibrium. You will only be defensive. Use peng jing and turn (your) waist and legs to neutralize the coming jing. *Taijiquan Classic* says: "If you fail to catch the opportunity and gain the superior position, (your) body will be disordered. To solve this problem, (you) must look to the waist and legs." Use the waist and the legs to find the neutralizing jing. Use the posture of peng to find central equilibrium. After long practice, the root will be firmed and the central equilibrium established.

其練法，由練伴拿我肘並尋我之中心，其意欲損我之中定也。我僅防守而不攻，以掤勁與腰腿轉化來勁。經云：〝有不得機得勢處，身便散亂。其病必於腰腿求之。〞此即其意也。由腰腿上，求化勁。由q勁勢上，尋中定。久而久之，根紮矣！中定矣！

In order to protect your central equilibrium, you need to keep your waist and hips loose. You must also know how to turn the waist to redirect the incoming force to the sides to neutralize. Zhang, San-Feng (張三豐) in his *Taijiquan Classic* has describes the importance of the waist and legs as an answer to becoming overcome by an opponent.

A good method of training this is to let your opponent control your elbows and put you in an urgent situation. Then you can use your waist and legs to neutralize the situation, rolling and directing the attack into emptiness. We will explore this exercise in chapter 2.

1.5 Yin and Yang, Insubstantial and Substantial

To become a proficient taijiquan practitioner in pushing hands training, you must know the yin and yang sides of taijiquan practice and how to apply these actions to gain an advantage in pushing hands training. The most fundamental aspect of taijiquan is its creation from the theory of yin and yang, including including its derivation from wuji, or no extremity. Understanding this concept will allow you to be able to cover the entire scope of training. In this section, we will explore this topic utilizing the following theses.

[Movements]: "When (it) moves, then (it) divides, when (it is) calm, it unites." "Dividing is the dividing of yin and yang, and the unification is the unification of yin and yang. The appearance of taijiquan is as such. Dividing and unifying are all applied to myself." "The opponent does not know me, only I know the opponent." This means understanding jing. After a long time of pondering, then you will comprehend automatically.[8]

《動》：〝動之則分，靜之則合。〞分為陰陽之分，合為陰陽之合，太極之形如此：分合皆謂己而言。〝人不知我，我獨知人〞，懂勁之謂也，揣摩日久自悉矣。

Here author Wǔ, Cheng-Qing (武澄清) offers his thoughts regarding movements of taijiquan. When you are calm and still, you are in the state of wuji (無極), or no extremity. Once you initiate the movements, you begin your journey of yin and yang separation. The whole concept of taijiquan arises from this notion.

If you have studied the classics you most likely have examined the works of taijiquan master Wang, Zong-Yue (王宗岳). He is well known for his description of taiji and its relationship to both the wuji state and yin and yang. From his explanation we are able to realize the true meaning of taiji and how the driving force of your mind is able to cause the division of yin and yang in the martial art of taijiquan. You will begin to understand the division and unification of such polarities and how they are applied in the actions of taijiquan. These physical manifestations of your mind's actions will also extend to your opponent and thus you will reach the goal of understanding yourself and your opponent.

There are few people who cultivate (the theory) of taiji's yin and yang. Ask for (i.e., demand) the hardness (i.e., yang) and softness (i.e., yin) in swallow (i.e., neutralize) and split (i.e., attack), open (i.e., extending), and close (i.e., storing). (If) the withdrawal and release of the four sides and four corners (can be) executed as you wish, (then) why should (you) worry about the variations of the movements and the calmness? (When) the production and the conquest two methods can be applied as desired, to dodge or to advance can all be found in the movements. How to apply the lightness and the heaviness in the insubstantial and substantial, (the key is) do not hesitate to manifest the light in the heaviness.[9]

太極陰陽少人修，吞吐開合問剛柔。

正隅收放任君走，動靜變化何須愁。

生剋二法隨著用，閃進全在動中求。

輕重虛實怎的是，重裡現輕勿稍留。

From the preceding passage Yang, Yu (Ban-Hou) (楊鈺) (班侯) speaks of the mind's intent to generate yin and yang within taijiquan. There are many who are content simply with the actions of taijiquan and few who spend the time pondering the depths of taiji's yin and yang. Remember, it is your mind that guides you from the wuji (no extremity) state to the yin-yang state and back. The separation of yin and yang also contains many levels of division. This training is a continuous process that leads one to the unconscious level of acting without thought or a state of regulating without regulating, thus having no hesitation in movement.

Practitioners of taijiquan training have five theories of training. All of these theories incorporate yin and yang elements. Whether you are cultivating the yin side of spiritual development or the yang side of martial training, those elements should be explored and understood before training pushing hands. If you wish to understand these theories further we highly recommend referring to the book, *Taijiquan Theory of Dr. Yang, Jwing-Ming*, as well as other taijiquan books offered by YMAA Publication Center.

Pushing hands provides training to expand the knowledge of yin-yang polarities beyond the self. You are now interacting with another force, exchanging yin and yang forces with the intent of disrupting your opponent's energy and causing them to lose their central equilibrium, all while maintaining your center and root. They in turn are also attempting to do the same things to you. The division of yin and yang will increase the possibilities.

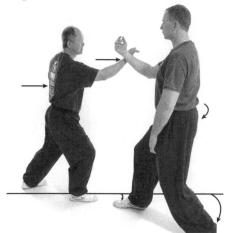
Defensive yang (step) and yin (deflect).

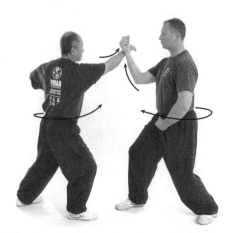
Defensive yin (no step) and yang (deflect).

The training develops an increase in awareness of the myriad layers of yin and yang and that there are multiple solutions generated from these layers. To further illustrate this concept, we will examine one situation. Keep in mind this example is merely highlighting a simple division of yin and yang.

Stand facing your opponent. They execute an attack toward you with their right hand (yang action). In defending the attack (yin action), you may either step to the right to intercept the opponent's right arm with your right hand or you may stay in place and deflect your opponent's right arm with your right arm. In the first situation you step to the side (yang action) and intercept the incoming force without deflecting its original intent of action (yin action). In the second situation you remain in place (yin action) and deflect the incoming force from its original intent of action (yang action). Keep in mind this is only one simple level of yin-yang division seen from the point of view of the defender and you should also realize that both defensive actions can be correct depending on the situation.

1.5.1 Insubstantial and Substantial (Xu, Shi, 虛、實)

When engaging an opponent for taiji pushing hands or engaging an opponent in fighting, one must have the knowledge of substantial and insubstantial. These two concepts are crucial to find the path to victory. Here we will introduce some basic theories related to substantial and insubstantial. For those of you who wish to explore more in depth we recommend you look to YMAA Publication Center for various books on this subject.

(The success of manifesting) insubstantial, insubstantial-substantial, and substantial (strategies) is (all hidden) in the meeting (i.e., gathering of concentration) of spirit. Insubstantial and substantial, substantial and insubstantial, the hands (are mainly used to) perform these achievements. (If) training fist (i.e., martial arts) without knowing the theory of insubstantial and substantial, (then) wasting gongfu and (the arts) will be completed at the end. Defense with insubstantial and attack with substantial, the tricky (keys) are in the palms. (If only) keep the center substantial without attacking, the art will be hard to refine. Insubstantial and substantial must have their reasons as the insubstantial and substantial. (If you know how to apply) insubstantial, insubstantial-substantial, and substantial, then the attack will not be in vain.[10]

虛虛實實神會中，虛實實虛手行功。

練拳不諳虛實理，枉費功夫終無成。

虛守實發掌中竅，中實不發藝難精。

虛實自有虛實在，實實虛虛攻不空。

From this passage Yang, Yu (Ban-Hou) (楊鈺) (班侯) teaches us that the concept of insubstantial is related to a fake action and is classified as yin while the real action or strategy is related to substantial and is known as a yang action. One must be familiar with these concepts or your opponent will be able to see your intent and easily defeat you. To be effective in this exchange your spirit must be high. When the spirit is high, alertness and awareness are high. This will lead to a more effective exchange between the strategies as well as a more timely response to your opponent's actions.

In taijiquan training you will mainly perform these actions with your hands. Your hands must develop a high sense of awareness, allowing you to feel your opponent's intentions. Once you have developed this high sense of awareness you will be able to execute your insubstantial and substantial actions more accurately.

1.6 Six Turning Secrets of Taijiquan

To become a proficient taijiquan pushing hands martial artist, you must also understand and be skillful in the six turning secrets of taijiquan. These are turning secrets are the crucial keys of entering a higher level of taijiquan martial skills. Without this knowledge you will not understand the basics of how the body and mind is able to transfer between yin and yang when encountering your opponent. The following is a summary of the six turning secrets.

Eight Doors and Five Steppings are the main essence and fundamental structures of taijiquan. From these Thirteen Postures, it (i.e., taijiquan) further evolved and resulted in the derivation of six living turning skills. They have since become the most important (essence) of taijiquan's pushing hands and sparring applications. If those who learn taijiquan can ponder and comprehend these six turning secrets thoroughly and apply them skillfully and with liveliness, then their achievement in taijiquan will surely reach the peak (of the art).

八門五步乃太極拳之主要精髓與基本結構。由此十三勢進而演繹出六個活用之轉動技巧，為太極拳推手與散打應用中之首要。學太極拳者，如能參透與澈底的去領悟此六轉訣並活用之，則其太極拳之造詣，必能登峰。

The entire art of taijiquan is constructed from thirteen basic actions. These thirteen actions are commonly called "Thirteen Postures" (shi san shi, 十三勢), which are constructed from the eight basic jing (勁) (i.e., power manifestation) patterns and five basic stepping strategies. Therefore, the Thirteen Postures are also commonly called the "Eight Doors" (ba men, 八門) and "Five Steppings" (wu bu, 五步). "Eight Doors" is used simply because from these basic eight jing patterns, the eight directions—including the four formal directions of front, rear, left, and right, and also the four diagonal corners—can be effectively protected and techniques can be executed.

In addition, the development of taijiquan is built upon the concepts of "round" and "circling" actions. With the Thirteen Postures and the concept of roundness, six turning secrets can be discerned. In fact, these six turning secrets are the most important fundamentals of taijiquan's pushing hands and free fighting applications. Taijiquan practitioners who are interested in taijiquan pushing hands and free sparring and who ponder, study, and practice these six turning secrets diligently can achieve a profound level of skill.

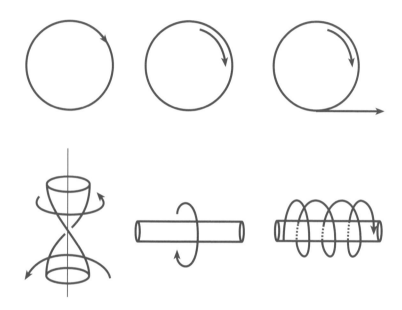

Six Turning Strategic Actions of Taijiquan.

What are the six turning secrets? They are circling, spinning, rotating, twisting, coiling, and spiraling. When circling is applied in the stepping, it is the living application of "Five Steppings." From the steadiness of "central equilibrium" (zhong ding), with the coordination of advancing forward, retreating backward, beware of the left, and looking to the right, the circle is formed through stepping. When the circling is used in the body's maneuvering, it is the circling (or half circling) of the touching hands that can thus be used to lead and neutralize (the coming power).

六轉訣者，圈轉、自轉、旋轉、扭轉、纏轉、與螺旋轉也。圈轉之用
於步伐，乃五步之活用。由中定之定，配合前進，後退、左顧、右盼
而成步圈。圈轉之用於身法，為八門搭手之輾轉〔半轉圈〕與引化。

Of the six turnings, circling is the largest action, and can be used for stepping or the body's maneuvering actions. From stepping-circling, you can enter the opponent's empty door (kong men, 空門), which can provide you with an opportunity for attack. In addition, through stepping-circling, you can evade the opponent's aggressive forward or sideways attack. In a fight, if you step in a straight line, it is easier for your opponent to follow you and to corner you. However, if you know how to step with a circling action skillfully, then it will be very difficult for your opponent to trap you in a corner.

The body's circling action initiates the arms' circling action. From the arms' circling, you can yield, lead, and then neutralize. In fact, the success of using "four ounces to repel a thousand pounds" relies on how skillfully you are able to circle your arms.

What is spinning? Under the conditions of "central equilibrium" and also the stillness of the axle, the body spins so as to neutralize the coming force. Spinning is just like the steering wheel of a car. Under the condition of stillness in the axle, the steering wheel can be turned clockwise or counterclockwise as wished. Consequently, the car wheel can be orientated in the desired direction. Where is the body's axle? It is our body's gravity center, the lower dan tian, the central (area) of the waist, and is the root of central equilibrium. From the stillness and equilibrium of this center, the waist is able to spin as wished, and (then the jing) can be manifested at the fingers. *Taijiquan Classic* says: "The root is at the feet, (jing or movement is) generated from the legs, mastered (i.e., controlled) by the waist, and manifested (i.e., expressed) from the fingers."

自轉者，乃在中定不變之下，由軸心不動之前題下，身體自轉以引化
來勢。自轉者，如開車之轉盤也。在軸心位置不移動之下，而轉盤可
順時、逆時針而轉動，車輪因而轉向自如。身體之軸心者，身體之重
心也，下丹田也，腰之中心也，中定之本根也。由此中定，腰之自轉
如意，而顯現於手指。太極拳經云：〝其根在腳，發於腿，主宰於
腰，形於手指。〞即此意也。

Spinning takes place without any movement of the center or axle—the edge is turning. In the human body, this center is the center of gravity where the real dan tian (zhen dan tian, 真丹田) is located. If you can stabilize this center, you will be able to reach the goal of central equilibrium (zhong ding, 中定) in taijiquan. In order to maintain this equilibrium, your waist area must be exceedingly soft, relaxed, and mobile. To reach this goal, your kua (胯) (i.e., hip joint area) must also be loose and soft. If your kua area is tensed, your waist will also be tensed and stiff.

The body's spinning is controlled by the waist and is the most important key to neutralizing incoming power and for jing manifestation. Those who know how to keep the waist area soft and use it efficiently should be able to lead and direct the incoming power easily.

What is rotating? It is turning while shifting position. That is, the body spins while the center of the body is moving. It is just like the wheel's spinning and the axle's moving. Thus, (the car) is able to roll forward, roll backward, roll to the left, and roll to the right. In taijiquan, under the condition of central equilibrium, the body rotates with the coordination of forward, backward, left, and right stepping actions. Consequently, the body is able to roll forward, roll backward, roll to the left, and roll to the right so as to lead and neutralize the coming force and also to set up tactics and maneuvers.

旋轉者，移轉也，亦即身體中心移動中之自轉也。如車輪之旋轉與輪軸心之移動，因而可轉進、轉退、滾左、滾右。太極拳中，在中定之下，身體之旋轉與進、退、左、右步伐之配合行動也。由此身體之轉進、轉退、滾左、滾右，以引化來勢，以定玄機也。

Rotating is different from spinning. In spinning, the center or the axle does not move. However, in rotating, the center or the axle is also moving while spinning. Since there is a shifting of the center, you can yield while at the same time neutralizing the incoming force through spinning. In fact, rotating is one of the keys to neutralizing and repositioning yourself in moving pushing hands and sparring. Rotating is also a key to neutralizing the opponent's elbow strike (zhou, 肘) or the opponent's bumping (kao, 靠) techniques.

Twisting refers to the twisting of the joints. From the twisting of the ankles, knees, and hips, the upper body can be spun and rotated, and can therefore lead and neutralize the coming force. From the twisting of the opponent's wrists, elbows, and shoulders, you can seize and control his joints. Furthermore, from the twisting of your own joints, you can store your jing and be ready to emit.

扭轉者，關節之扭轉也。由足、膝、胯關節之扭轉產生上身之自轉與旋轉，因而可引化彼之來勢。由腕、肘、肩關節之扭轉，我可擒拿扣制彼方之關節。更由我關節之扭轉，我勁得以蓄積，待之而發。

Most of the twisting actions in taijiquan are in the joint areas. The body's spinning and rotating actions are initiated from the twisting of the three leg joints. If these three joints can be twisted and controlled carefully and efficiently, you will be able to keep your upper body upright and centered. In addition, the firmness of the root is determined by how soft and how flexible you keep these three joints as well. From this, you can see that the neutralization efficacy of the body is decided by the flexibility and mobility of your leg joints. Not only that, many jings are stored through the leg's twisting position. Note that you should train the knee areas especially with extreme care. Your goal is to encourage opening, strength, and flexibility of the joint, and not to push it to its limits.

When you apply the twisting action to the three joints of your arms, you can seize and control (i.e., qin na, 擒拿) the opponent's joints. In the same manner as with the leg's joints, through twisting, you can store jing in the arms.

> In coiling, you use (your) hands to coil around the opponent's arm so as to exchange the yin and yang (maneuvers). Consequently, the opponent's joints can be positioned under your palms for your control. Furthermore, from coiling, you can open your opponent's skylight (tian chuang) and ground window (di hu) for your use. What is spiraling? It means coiling forward or backward. From spiraling, you can coil the opponent's arm and move from one joint to another joint, which could therefore prevent the opponent from escaping. This is the proficient level of na jing (i.e., controlling jing) in taijiquan pushing hands training.

> 纏轉者，以手纏繞彼臂，以變陰、陽。因而，彼之關節可在我掌下，而為我所拿。甚之，由纏轉中，我可開彼之天窗、地戶而為我所趁。螺旋轉者，在纏轉中而進、退也。由螺旋轉，我可由纏轉彼臂自一關節而至另一關節，而不讓彼輕易逃脫。此為太極推手拿勁訓練之高層次也。

Coiling in taijiquan means to coil your hand around the opponent's arm like a snake coiling around a branch. This coiling action allows you to change the yin to yang and vice versa. For example, if your wrist is under the opponent's palm, you will be in a defensive and disadvantageous situation (i.e., yin situation). If you know the skill of coiling you will be able to coil around his wrist and position your hand above his wrist and thus change your defensive and disadvantageous situation into a favorable one (i.e., yang situation). In addition, through coiling action, you will be able to open the area above his arms (i.e., sky window) (tian chuang, 天窗) or under his armpit area (i.e., ground wicket) (i.e., di hu, 地戶) for attack.

Spiraling is slightly different from coiling. Spiraling refers to moving forward or backward while coiling. It is just like a snake that wraps around a branch and moves forward. In taijiquan, this skill allows you to move from one joint to another. In fact, coiling and spiraling are the two major keys of the na jing (拿勁) (i.e., controlling jing) in taijiquan pushing hands and sparring.

With the above six turning secrets, yin and yang can be exchanged skillfully in three dimensions. This is the crucial secret in pushing hands and sparring (training). They allow (you) to change a disadvantageous situation into an advantageous situation, to attack or defend as wished, and to put the opponent in a confused and dazed condition. The opponent does not know you; however, you know the opponent. To reach the proficiency of these six turning secrets, (you) must practice yin-yang taiji circle coiling, searching for clear comprehension, skillfulness, and their living applications. Those who practice taijiquan should ponder them carefully.

由上六轉訣，陰陽可互變在三度空間中，為推手、散打之要訣。可轉逆勢於順勢，可攻、可守如意自由，可置敵於恍惚之中。敵不知我，我卻知敵。此六轉訣，為能順手，必由太極圈纏手中去練習，求慎解、熟練、與活用。習太極拳者，應慎思之。

If taijiquan practitioners wish to seriously study and understand the essence of taijiquan martial applications, they must first ponder, comprehend, and practice the skills of these six turning secrets in three dimensions. The ancient taijiquan master, Li, Yi-She (李亦畬), said: "In the insubstantial, (the techniques) vary following the opportunity (i.e., situation). The marvelous (tricks) are found in the round." Roundness is the key to the six turning secrets.

References

1. Dr. Yang, Jwing-Ming, *Tai Chi Secrets of the Yang Style* (太極拳楊氏先哲祕要) (Wolfeboro, NH: YMAA Publication Center, 2001), 167.

2. Dr. Yang, Jwing-Ming, *Tai Chi Secrets of the Wu Style* (太極拳吳氏先哲祕要) (Wolfeboro, NH: YMAA Publication Center, 2002), 51.

3. Dr. Yang, Jwing-Ming, *Tai Chi Secrets of the Wǔ and Li Style* (太極拳武、李氏先哲祕要) (Wolfeboro, NH: YMAA Publication Center, 2001), 57.

4. Dr. Yang, Jwing-Ming, *Tai Chi Secrets of the Wu Style (*太極拳吳氏先哲祕要*)*, 5.

5. Dr. Yang, Jwing-Ming, *Tai Chi Secrets of the Wǔ and Li Style* (太極拳武、李氏先哲祕要), 61.

6. Dr. Yang, Jwing-Ming, *Tai Chi Secrets of the Wu Style* (太極拳吳氏先哲祕要), 26.

7. Dr. Yang, Jwing-Ming, *Tai Chi Secrets of the Yang Style* (太極拳楊氏先哲祕要), 50.

8. Dr. Yang, Jwing-Ming, *Tai Chi Secrets of the Wǔ and Li Style* (太極拳武、李氏先哲祕要), 23.

9. Dr. Yang, Jwing-Ming, *Tai Chi Secrets of the Yang Style* (太極拳楊氏先哲祕要), 26.

10. Dr. Yang, Jwing-Ming, *Tai Chi Secrets of the Yang Style* (太極拳楊氏先哲祕要), 22.

Chapter 2: Taiji Qigong Practice—Foundation

2.1 Introduction

The following section introduces you to some of the basic exercises necessary for training the mind and body for pushing hands practice. We introduce you to various methods of rooting, centering, grand circulation, taiji ball, and taiji yin-yang symbol training. Each exercise has multiple stages. Most exercises, if not all, end with training with the eyes closed. Be sure to complete each stage before going on to the next. The importance of training these exercises have been discussed in countless taiji classics written by various masters. You must learn to find your root, find your center, open the joints, and train the waist to be loose in order to maintain your balance. Without learning how to find your center and how to redirect incoming forces you will be unable to remain focused and will be easily defeated.

2.2 Rooting

We touched upon the theory of rooting in chapter 1. We cannot emphasize enough the importance of having a strong root when encountering an opponent. Without it, jing manifestation will be shallow, your mind will float, and the spirit will be shallow. In addition, your opponent will be able to uproot you more easily. In this section we discuss the training exercises to increase your awareness and depth of rooting beginning with lower root training then continuing to the middle section. Other exercises will include push-pull training and centering training with a partner.

1. Lower Section Body Gong (Rooting) (Xia Pan Gong-Ding Gen, 下盤功-定根)

The first exercise for root training is to stand in the ma bu (馬步) stance. Ma bu means horse stance and resembles the posture your body would assume while riding a horse. Remain in this stance for five minutes. Gradually extend the time you remain in the stance in five minute increments until you are able to remain in the stance comfortably for at least an hour.

While you are in ma bu, you may also practice reverse abdominal breathing techniques.

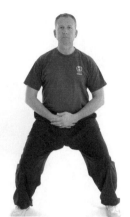

Stand with your legs slightly wider than shoulder width apart. The feet should be parallel to each other. Bend the knees and squat down until you are half way between an upright position and a full squat position in which the thighs are parallel to the ground. Your knees should be vertically aligned with your feet. Remain in this position for a minimum of five minutes.

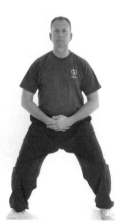

Place your hands over the lower dan tian area, your left hand over your right hand. Begin the reverse abdominal breathing technique while keeping your mind focused six inches below the surface on which you are standing. Each time you exhale, squat slightly to assist the mind in leading qi through the surface.

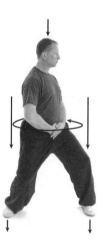

Once you have built up your ability to stand in the ma bu for thirty minutes, add a twisting of the body to both the left and right. Exhale each time you twist to the left or the right. Inhale as you return to the forward facing position. This will further strengthen the joints of the ankles, knees, and hips.

Continue to train this exercise daily until you are able to perform the exercise with twisting for a minimum of thirty minutes with no discomfort.

Next, begin brick training. Brick training increases the distance below the surface your mind will have to focus. Standing on bricks also creates a smaller area to stand on and will decrease the size of the focal point.

Begin brick training with the bricks on their sides (low), and then straight up and down (tall), followed by standing on bricks stacked on top of each other.

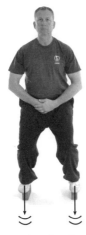
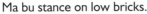

Ma bu stance on low bricks.

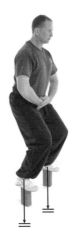

Ma bu stance on tall bricks.

Of course, standing on bricks can be very dangerous and we caution you to take your time before progressing from one level to the next. It is important to be comfortable enough to be able to move the body and practice jing patterns before attempting to train on two and three bricks.

Tips to Avoid Common Errors. The common errors that occur while standing in the ma bu position mainly are improper alignment of the legs as well as pushing the waist backward too far or bending over while squatting down. When positioning yourself in the ma bu stance you should keep the knees vertically aligned with the feet. This especially holds true for beginners when twisting from side to side. This will keep the force applied to the joints more of a twisting action than a medial/lateral force that could lead to injury. Additionally, one should tilt the hips forward slightly while squatting to allow the waist to be in a neutral position while standing in the ma bu position. This allows the spine to be in a more natural state and will allow the body to relax, leading to more efficient circulation of qi.

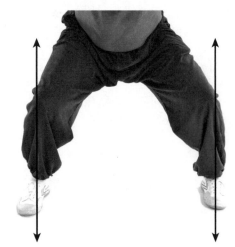

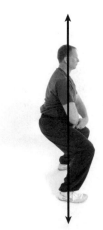

Ma bu stance knees correct.   Ma bu stance correct hips.

2. Circle Lower Section (Xia Pan Zhuan Quan, 下盤轉圈)

The next exercise for lower section training is circling lower section training. The purpose of this exercise is to increase the range of motion in the joints of the ankles, knees, and hips by shifting and twisting the body while in a squatted position. This action will also increase the flow of qi throughout the legs and strengthen the area.

The knees should be vertically aligned with the feet in the initial stance. Once the circling action is initiated, the knees will also begin making small circles over the feet. As you continue to shift your weight back and forth while circling, there will be a slight increase in the lateral and medial force on the collateral ligaments of the knee. Please note, it is important to start with the ma bu training. Ma bu training builds the strength of the ligaments necessary to prevent injury.

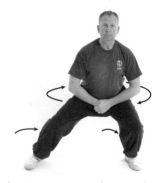

To begin this exercise, stand in a wide ma bu stance and squat down to a relatively low position. The lower the stance the more intense the training will be on your tendons, ligaments, and muscles. However, you should always begin training at a height comfortable for you in order to avoid injury. Begin to circle the waist either clockwise or counterclockwise while shifting your weight back and forth.

Continue this action for twelve repetitions then repeat, circling and twisting the waist in the opposite direction for the same number of repetitions.

The next stage of the lower circling section is done while standing on bricks. Extreme caution should be taken when practicing this exercise on bricks. When you shift your weight from one side to the other, there is a tendency to push off to the sides, which will cause you to fall.

Practice this exercise for twelve repetitions in both directions. Be sure to include twisting the waist in both directions. For the final stage, practice this exercise with your eyes closed.

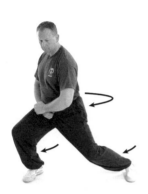

Continue to circle your waist in the desired direction then begin to twist the waist in the direction toward which you are shifting the weight.

Tips to Avoid Common Errors. The most common errors concern alignment of your knees. Initially, you will want to keep the knees relatively lined up with your feet. As you continue to circle your legs, you will increase the circling of the knees over your ankles. Do not allow the knees to fold inward while doing the exercise. Although there are more fibers in the medial side of the knee for handing increased loads, the exercise is designed for twisting and opening the joints. Avoid sticking your butt out or bending over while circling. Bending over not only will shift the weight too far backward but will make it easier for you to close your legs inward, thus defeating the object of opening the joints. The upper body needs to stay in a vertical posture. Otherwise you will lose your center and it will become easier for your opponent to uproot you. Additionally, make sure you twist your waist in the direction you turn your body. Your waist is the director of power. Turning the waist will help loosen the hip joints up so that you keep that area alive. Doing so allows you to redirect power both outbound and inbound.

3. Middle Section Body Gong—Loosening the Waist and Kua (Song Yao, Song Kua, 鬆腰，鬆胯)

This exercise focuses on training two areas in the middle section of the body. The first area is known as the kua (胯) or hip joint. The second area is the lumbar section of the spine. From *Taijiquan Classic*: "The root is at the feet, (jing or movement is) generated from the legs, mastered (i.e., controlled) by the waist, and manifested (i.e., expressed) from the fingers. From the feet to the legs to the waist must be integrated, and one unified qi. When moving forward or backward, (you can) catch the opportunity and gain the superior position."[1] Zhang, San-Feng (張三豐) is saying the waist is a major factor in directing the manifestation of power. In order to direct this power the waist must be open and strong. This exercise will assist in this.

To practice this exercise, step into a ma bu stance. The right hand will be placed on the lower dan tian area while the left hand will be placed on the sacrum, palm facing away from the body. Imagine the tailbone is a writing utensil and you will be using it to draw a circle on the ground between your legs. Start circling the waist in a counterclockwise direction. Begin with small circles and continue to increase each one until you have reached a comfortable range of motion. Focus the action on the movement of the lumbar section of the spine. Inhale while circling around the backside of the body and exhale while circling around the forward side of the

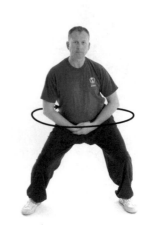

Ma bu circle exercise for waist and kua.

body. Repeat the circling action for twelve repetitions. Next, twist the body to the right while horizontally circling the waist. Continue to twist in that direction until you reach the point where you are no longer able to keep the original size of your circle. Complete twelve more repetitions then twist the body toward the opposite direction. Repeat the circling action while facing left. Finally, twist back to the forward-facing position and decrease the circling action of the waist until you have arrived at the starting point. Once you have reached this position, begin to circle the waist horizontally in a clockwise direction. Continue to circle the waist for twelve repetitions while facing forward as well as to the right and left. You will twist to the left and right only as far as you are able without causing discomfort and sacrificing the original size of your circle. To end this training exercise simply turn back to the facing forward position and decrease the circling action until reaching the starting point.

The next stage of this exercise follows the same sequence of the stationary ma bu training with the additional challenge of standing on bricks. To start, place the bricks on their sides while practicing the horizontal circling action of the waist. Once you are comfortable on the sideway bricks, place the bricks in the upright position. Repeat the exercise for each of the directions until you are comfortable. In the next stage, add another brick on either side and repeat the exercise until you are comfortable. Individuals who are able to perform this exercise comfortably while standing on three or more bricks are considered to have a strong root with a flexible waist.

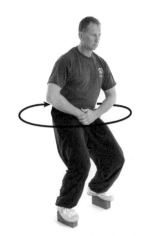

Ma bu circle exercise on low bricks for waist and kua.

Tips to Avoid Common Errors. The most common error when performing these exercises relates to the circling of the waist and swaying or shifting the weight back and forth between the legs. It is incorrect to sway or shift back and forth. The purpose of the exercise is to focus on the lower section of your spine and waist. You are attempting to keep the body relatively upright and the weight evenly distributed between the feet. When you circle the waist you will want to tilt the hips left and right as well as forward and back in order to make the circling action. Although not completely necessary, it is a good idea to vertically align the knees over the feet initially. This will help train the hips to open up, especially when you twist the body to either side.

Twisting the Sand Bag (Niu Zhuan Sha Dai, 扭轉沙袋)

These exercises involve a hanging heavy bag or sand bag, the kind often used for punching or kicking. This type of training assists the mind in partner training and in the manifestation of power. It helps you develop a firm root and manifest this power through the whole body.

To begin, stand in front of the training bag in the ma bu stance.

Place your hands on the bag then twist your body back and forth while maintaining a wardoff (peng, 掤) posture throughout the whole body. The hands will move back and forth horizontally, which in turn will cause the training bag to twist back and forth. Each time you twist your body, sink into your legs. Initially, your hands will be placed on the bag at waist height. After you are comfortable with this action, raise your hands higher while twisting your body.

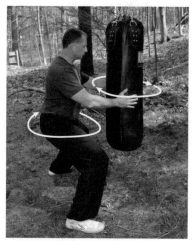

Heavy bag twisting exercise.

Next, practice by twisting your waist back and forth while striking the sides of the bag. One palm will strike the side of the bag at approximately the same height as your face. The other palm will strike the opposite side of the bag approximately the same height as the dan tian area. This will be followed by twisting your body and attacking the bag diagonally with the palms of your hands. For each twisting action, one palm will strike the bag diagonally forward at approximately the same height as your face. The opposite palm will strike the bag diagonally toward your body at approximately dan tian height. Continue these movements until you have repeated this exercise for twelve repetitions for each angle.

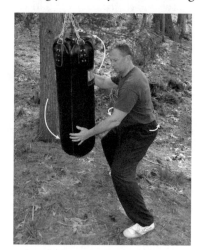

Heavy bag twisting exercise with striking.

Tips to Avoid Common Errors. The most common errors involve connecting the body with the arms. The movement needs to be from the whole body, not just the arms. Pay attention to your waist, and follow through the hands. Additionally, the arms move in unison. This means the attacking occurs simultaneously with both hands striking the bag. When you twist the bag horizontally, the action is simultaneous, with one hand moving forward and the other moving backward. In the diagonal drill, one hand moves up and forward while the other moves down and back. Finally, you must pay attention to sinking the body when attacking the bag. Over time this action will become instinctual and occur more naturally

4. Bumping (Kao, 靠)

Bumping, or kao, is one of the Thirteen Postures contained within the movements of taijiquan. This action can be executed using your chest, back, leg, and in some cases even your head. It can be used to either strike an opponent in places such as the solar plexus or used to bounce or throw an opponent, thus uprooting them.

(When) stepping forward to use kao (i.e., bump) strike, it is as competing with a swimming dragon. (When) kao is used, the leg straightly (i.e., directly) enters the opponent's crotch. (When striking) from the bottom to the top, turn the body urgently. (Use) the shoulder to strike the opponent's chest; do not show mercy. Absolutely do not (use) single leg to support the body (i.e., center), which allows the opponent the space to withdraw. Kao strike is frequently varied from the cai. (When) the opponent dodges (my bump), I use pluck to accomplish my technique.

進步打靠賽游龍。靠腿直入敵襠中。

由下斜上急轉身，肩打敵胸不容情。

切忌一腿不鼎主，致使對方有餘容。

靠打多由採手變，敵閃我採招法成。

Taijiquan master Li, Yi-She refers to the use of kao as resembling a swimming dragon when attacking an opponent. One must be fluid in nature and act swiftly, closing the distance by entering into the opponent's crotch area with your legs. When executing this jing, remain centered and rooted. The action begins from the feet and is done quickly so the opponent doesn't have the chance to withdraw. If they withdraw you may use cai or pluck to assist in your bumping technique.

How do we explain the bump jing (kao jing)? Its techniques are divided into shoulders and back. Diagonal flying uses the shoulder, and within the (application of the) shoulder, there also is a back. Once gaining the advantageous position, (bump the opponent) with a deafening sound like a pounding pestle. Be careful to keep the weighting center, (if) losing it, the effort will be in vain.

靠勁義何解，其法分肩背。

斜飛勢用肩，肩中還有背。

一旦得機勢，轟然如搗碓。

仔細維重心，失中徒無功。

Here Wu, Gong-Zao further illustrates the use of bumping while using the diagonal flying movement in the taijiquan sequence. As in the taijiquan pushing hands exercises this action emphasizes the use of the shoulders or back for attacking. He also stresses the need for being centered and applying the technique forcefully and without hesitation.

In the following exercises we will demonstrate only the bumping actions using your shoulder. Although we are training the precursor to martial applications, we are focusing on the use of bumping techniques in taijiquan pushing hands. The most common areas used in this attack are the shoulders and back.

In this next exercise, bump the bag from behind your body.

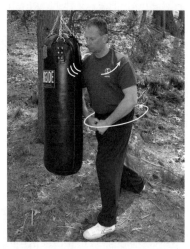

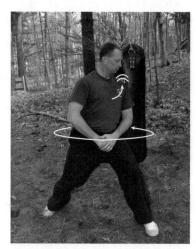

To practice the first exercise, stand in front of the bag. Twist your body in either direction and strike the bag with your shoulder. As you apply your bumping action to the bag, sink into your feet. Once you have struck the bag, immediately twist your body back to the original position. Practice this exercise for at least twelve times for each side.

Stand facing away from the bag then twist your body in either direction to strike the bag with the back of your body. Once you have made contact, immediately return to your starting position. Repeat this exercise for at least twelve times for each side.

Tips to Avoid Common Errors. Common errors related to this exercise include overreaching or bending the body over to attack the bag. You need to be close enough to the bag to properly make contact with the bag. There is also a tendency to twist the waist, make contact with the bag, and remain in that position while the bag sways forward then back, making contact with your body for the second time. Due to the nature of the kao posture, you should strike and return the body back to the original position. From there you may reapply your kao action if you wish to immediately repeat the movement.

5. Arcing the Arms or Embracing the Moon on the Chest (Gong Shou, 拱手; Hui Zhong Bao Yue, 懷中抱月)

The original name for this exercise is the Three Power Posture (San Cai Shi, 三才勢). It relates to the connection of heaven, man, and earth and the flow of this particular path of qi. It is a common exercise for the beginner who wishes to experience qi. It is also an important tool for a taiji practitioner who is planning to engage in taiji pushing hands. In its advanced training, an individual learns to build qi not only in the shoulders but through two additional qi circuits. One path is vertical and runs from your baihui cavity (Gv-20) (百會) on the top of your head, down the spine to the lower dan tian, then out the yongquan cavity (K-1) (湧泉) into the earth. The second path is horizontal and runs from the chest out the shoulders along the arms to the hands and back to the chest. Through the continued training of circulating the qi smoothly throughout these two paths, a practitioner will be able to build their qi to a higher level and increase their sensitivity or listening jing skills. In addition, the training will increase the strength of their body for the endurance of pushing hands training.

To practice this exercise, step into the false stance (xuan ji bu, 玄機步) (xu bu, 虛步). Raise your arms out in front of your body approximately chest height, forming a large horizontal circle. The hands should be close to each other but not touching. The back should be slightly rounded and the chest sunk. Allow the tongue to lightly touch the roof of the mouth in order to connect the conception and governing vessels. Begin to breathe deeply. Your mind should be calm and relaxed while you begin to lead the qi.

In the beginning, practice by focusing on one path at a time. For the vertical path, inhale and lead the qi into the baihui cavity and down into the lower dan tian. While exhaling, lead

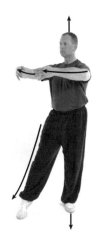

Arching the Arms or Embracing the Moon on the Chest.

the qi down and out your yongquan cavity. For the horizontal path you will lead the qi from the fingertips to the center of your chest on inhaling. When you exhale, lead the qi out from your chest to the fingertips and across the space between the hands. Hold this position for at least three minutes then switch the forward leg to the opposite one. Now hold this position for an additional three minutes while practicing your breathing techniques and qi circulation.

Keep in mind that the goal is to lead the qi in the two paths simultaneously. Through continued practice, you will be able to circulate your qi through both paths simultaneously. Over time you will want to increase the amount of time in this posture.

Tips to Avoid Common Errors. Common errors occur most often in how you hold your arms in front of the body. Relax the neck and do not shrug the shoulders. Shrugging the shoulders causes tension in the neck. This will result in trapping the qi in this area. To correct this, keep the arms out in front of the body no higher than the shoulders.

6. Push and Pull Rooting Training (Tui La Zha Gen Lian Xi, 推拉紮根練習)

Rooting practice with a partner through the game of tug of war. That means you and your partner stand in mountain climbing stance and face each other, the front hands holding each other (like a handshake). During competition, both sides try their best to pull the opponent off balance (in any direction). When there is any shift in rooting, then the one who shifts his root loses. From this practice, (you) can master the skills of leading and neutralizing the coming jing, to see clearly and to feel the opponent's central equilibrium and root. After practicing for a long time, the root can be firmed. The students should ponder, comprehend, and practice this game and catch its key tricks.[2]

與友伴練習紮根之法，可以拉拒戰行之。亦即與友伴蹬山步對立，前手相握。比賽時，盡力想將對方拉倒。根一動即敗。在此練習下，可熟悉如何將來勁引化，可洞悉感覺對方之中定與根源，久而久之，根定矣。學者當自習之以悟其竅。

The next set of exercises involve rooting training with a partner. You are testing the depth of each other's root.

To begin this exercise, face your partner with your right legs forward. Squat down into four-six stance (si liu bu, 四六步) and pluck your partner's right hand with your right hand. Attempt to uproot each other by pulling or pushing your partner's arm back and forth, causing them to become unbalanced.

Although you are plucking your partner's hand, you are focusing your mind down into his center and attempting to create an urgency in his mind to keep centered and rooted. This will entail shifting back and forth between four-six stance (si liu bu, 四六步) and mountain climbing stance (deng shan bu, 登山步)

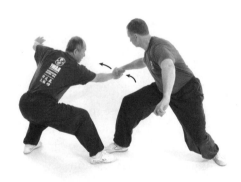

Rooting training with a partner. First stage: practice with feet on the ground.

while attempting to uproot your partner. Continue to practice this exercise until one of you has become unbalanced and falls away from their stance. Step back into the stance and practice the exercise again. Continue this practice until you are both comfortable then practice the exercise with the left leg forward.

The next stage of this exercise is to practice while on bricks. We cannot emphasize enough the amount of care you should take when training on bricks.

Place the bricks on the ground and on their sides, spacing them so you and your partner can stand on them with right legs forward. Again, grasp your partner's hand and begin to shift back and forth between mountain climbing (deng shan bu, 登山步) and four-six stances (si liu bu, 四六步) while attempting to uproot each other. Your mind will need to focus deeper into the ground to maintain your root while simultaneously searching further into your partner's center to uproot them.

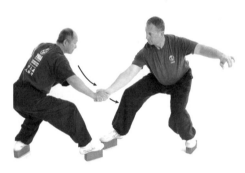

Be careful not to lean over when shifting back and forth between stances. This will create more opportunity for your partner to find your center and force your mind to float while attempting to regain your balance. Where your mind floats so too will the body, which will result in you falling off the bricks. Continue to practice this exercise until you are both comfortable with maintaining your root

Second stage: practice while standing on bricks.

on the bricks. Also practice the same exercise on the bricks with the left leg forward. Of course, after you both are able, you may continue to deepen the training by placing the bricks upright as well as stacking bricks on top of one another. The final stage is performing the exercise with eyes closed.

Tips to Avoid Common Errors. Common errors tend to be related to leaning over too far and not connecting your waist to the movements. You need to keep yourself in an upright posture while shifting back and forth between stances. As your partner pushes into your root you need to twist your waist to redirect the force and return your attack. Wang, Zong-Yue (王宗岳) wrote, "Stand like a balanced scale, (move) lightly like a cartwheel."[3] Your body must be like a scale balancing weights. You need to remain in an upright position, centered, and in equilibrium. When you neutralize the incoming forces you must move the whole body in unison.

2.3 Centering (Central Equilibrium)

Centering training is one of the most important training tools to develop. Of the Thirteen Postures it is considered the second most important posture in taijiquan training. In taijiquan pushing hands training, the key is to find your center of gravity and keep this area loose in order to not be uprooted. This location is in the real dan tian (zhen dan tian, 真丹田) (i.e., center of gravity). During pushing hands training, your partner will seek out this area to uproot you and scatter your mind. To maintain your central equilibrium, you must be able to maintain the balance and stability of this real dan tian. You must be able to turn the waist and redirect the incoming energy to neutralize the force.

In chapter 2 we discussed various theories of central equilibrium and its relationship to pushing hands training. Here we will discuss exercises to assist in training your central equilibrium skills. The purpose of the following exercises is to yield to an incoming force and redirect that incoming force while maintaining your root and central equilibrium. You will also learn to adhere, stick, and follow the energy as it is withdrawn all while maintaining your central equilibrium.

In the first exercise you and your partner practice to become more familiar with your own center. You both also learn the feeling of how to yield to an incoming force as well as how to stick to the other person's force when they withdraw their attack. The purpose of this exercise is to learn to yield to the incoming force and to stay attached to the person as they withdraw their attack.

To train this first exercise, face your partner with right legs forward. Your partner will place either their right or left hand on various sections of your body such as the shoulders, waist area, or the center of your chest and push on that area. You will then yield to the incoming force by twisting your body and applying wardoff (peng, 掤). This action is known as swallowing. Swallowing occurs when you allow the incoming force to come in and be led into neutralization. At some point, your partner will no longer apply their attacking force and will begin to withdraw that hand. You will follow the movement back to the neutral position and await the next incoming force. As you become more comfortable with this action, have your partner increase the pace at which they push your body. Switch legs and practice the movements again. Next, change the offensive and defensive actions with your partner so they may also train the yielding action.

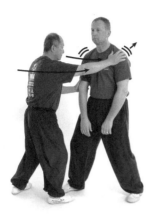 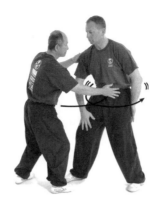 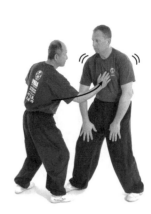

Centering training.

As you both become more comfortable, you and your partner will train the same exercise while standing on bricks. We recommend you start with the bricks flat and progress to higher positions only when you are both comfortable with each stage of the exercises.

Finally, you and your partner will practice this exercise while your eyes are closed.

Tips to Avoid Common Errors. Common errors often occur in the application of wardoff (peng, 掤) while yielding to the incoming force. You need to round out your back while creating the open area in front of your body. Be careful not to lean over while doing this. Also, remember this action is alive and applied as the force is felt upon your body. You must also focus on sticking with your partner when they retract the incoming force. This action is similar to being stuck to fly paper. When you close your eyes be careful not to lower your head. This occasionally causes the

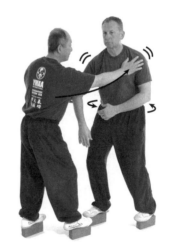

Centering training, standing on bricks.

body to lean forward and you will not be centered. Keep the chin tucked in and lift your head. Remember that you want to have the feeling of being pulled up by the top of the head. The waist also needs to be alive, meaning you must twist the waist back and forth while following the incoming force and following the withdrawal of the attack.

The next exercise is also a centering training. Once again you and your partner are attempting to find each other's center and uproot the other person before they uproot you. This exercise also incorporates the jing pattern known as controlling jing we describe in full under section 3-6. If you wish to use this movement in centering, we encourage you to read that section then work on the exercise presented here.

To practice centering training, face your partner with the right legs forward. Your stance will be narrow and high. Attach to each other's arms with your hands. Initially one person will attempt to find the other's center by pushing into any limb or body part. The idea is to find the center of gravity and uproot your partner, moving them from their fixed position on the ground. It is similar to finding the hinge of a door and pushing into it. The other person who is being attacked will attempt to redirect the incoming force or, as in our door example, change the location of the hinge of the door. In order to do so, first apply wardoff (peng, 掤) and turn the waist to redirect the

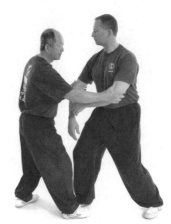

Centering training incorporating the jing pattern.

incoming force. On the first few attempts, practice this action slowly. Once you are more comfortable with the redirection of energy, you may increase the force and speed. Practice the exercise until the movements are smooth and controlled. Next, you and your partner will exchange the attacking and neutralizing sides. Practice this action again until it is continuous and smooth. Finally, you and your partner will practice the action back and forth, exchanging attacking and neutralizing simultaneously. Again, begin slowly then increase the force and speed. Practice this exercise until you both are able to maintain your center while the opposite person attacks from different angles.

The next stage of practicing centering is to train while standing on bricks. Be extra careful while performing this exercise on bricks and progress to higher brick positions only when you are both comfortable doing so. The final stage of this exercise is to practice it with your eyes closed.

Tips to Avoid Common Errors. There are many common errors to look for while practicing this particular exercise. The most common error is the improper use of wardoff jing (peng jing, 掤勁). Remember to use peng when an attack is incoming. Once the attack has been neutralized, peng jing may be released. Also, do not lean over when applying peng. The tailbone must be sunk and your head and body kept upright, otherwise you will find yourself off balance and your opponent may use the opportunity to change the direction of attack, resulting in you being uprooted. It is written, "When the body's shape, waist, and the crown of the head are all regulated correctly, the yi (i.e., wisdom mind) and the qi in attaching, adhering, connecting, and the following will be uniform (i.e., smooth)."[4] To execute these skills effectively, maintain an upright posture to keep your center and allow your spirit to be raised. You also must remain loose throughout the exercise. You must relax, or your opponent will be able to find your center easier. Avoid looking down. Keep your gaze forward toward your partner. Looking downward creates a tendency to lean over and you will find yourself off balance more often. When you and your partner are exchanging attacks and neutralizing, you must be careful of focusing on one side. This occurs when you are using only one hand at a time. You should think in terms of the whole body moving as one unit. An example of this is where you find yourself neutralizing an incoming attack with one arm and simultaneously attacking with the other arm. Always be aware of both sides. Finally, you must be aware of not overextending yourself when attacking your opponent. There is a temptation to continue the offensive attack beyond your range. This condition is known as butting.

> Butting means having overdone it (i.e., oversufficiency). Deficiency means not enough. Losing means separating. Resistance means (using) excessive force (to respond to the incoming force). (You) must know that the defaults of these four words are originated from not knowing attaching, adhering, connecting, and following. (If you are so), then it is certain that (you) do not know (how to apply) conscious feelings in actions. (When you) just learn how to match (i.e., spar) with the opponent, (you) must not without knowing these defaults. Furthermore, (you) must not (proceed) without getting rid of these defaults. (The reasons) why it is so difficult (to learn the skills) of attaching, adhering, connecting, and following is because it is not easy to avoid the butting, deficiency, losing, and resistance.[5]

> 頂者，出頭之謂也。匾者，不及之謂也。丟者，離開之謂也。抗者，太過之謂也。要知于此四字之病，不但粘、黏、連、隨，斷不明知覺運動也。初學對手，不可不知也。更不可不去此病。所難者，粘、黏、連、隨，而不許頂、匾、丟、抗是所不易矣。

Yang, Yu (Ban-Hou) (楊鈺) (班侯) explains the concept of overextending yourself, or "butting," in this selection. Overextending yourself will allow your opponent to use this force against you and unbalance you. Master Yang further describes other faults of pushing hands skills such as deficiency, losing, and resistance. All of these are caused by not knowing and training the basics of attaching, adhering, connecting, and following. You must train these skills in order to shed bad habits, otherwise you will remain very shallow in your training.

2.4 Heng and Ha Sounds Qigong

Within the martial community there are many different sounds that are used for practice and fighting. Those of you who train taijiquan have two important sounds that serve several purposes. These sounds are heng (哼) and ha (哈). Use of such sounds will assist you in emitting or withdrawing your jing to a maximum while coordinating your qi with the manifestation of the jing. Additionally, you will learn to raise your Spirit of Vitality. In the taiji classics it is written, "Grasp and hold the dan tian to train internal gongfu. Heng, ha two qi's are marvelous and infinite."[6] It is also written, "The Throat is the second master."[7] There also are a number of classics written with regard to lifting or suspending the head to raise the spirit. Keeping the spirit raised and focused will allow you to respond to your opponent's actions in a light and agile manner. Your qi will flow more naturally and become stronger. The use of these sounds will provide you with the necessary means of condensing and emitting your jing to a maximum. Finally, emitting such a sound will cause alarm to your opponent, possibly even causing a major distraction and giving you an advantage while engaging the person.

In the following paragraphs we will describe a few exercises to practice the sounds of heng and ha. After you have completed these exercises you will have a better understanding of this manifestation and you may apply these sounds to the other jing patterns described in other sections of this book. You may also begin to utilize these sounds while practicing your pushing hands drills.

Regardless of the sound, the manifestation should be made from deep within the body and not from the mouth. If not done properly, you will find your throat will become dry and sore quickly. To create these sounds, begin by drawing air from deep within the lungs. The sound will be then created in the vocal chords. This area also contains a cavity known to the Chinese as the tiantu (Co-22) (天突) cavity. It is known as the gate of expression, and its energy is balanced with another cavity known as the yintang (M-HN-3) (印堂) cavity. The yintang cavity is where the spirit resides. Furthermore, the tiantu cavity is paired with the dazhui cavity and as such is linked to the emotional mind, providing assistance in raising up the spirit. A raised spirit will cause the energy manifestation to be strong as well enhance awareness of your surroundings. Each of these sounds will be used in conjunction with reverse abdominal breathing. This type of breathing is related to physical manifestation and emotion. It is assumed that you are familiar with the different stages of breathing exercises. These techniques are common to the internal arts and are necessary for advanced stages of training.

There are two ways of manifesting the heng (哼) sound. The first way is purely yin in nature and is made while inhaling. It is very similar to the sound someone might make when they are suddenly frightened. While making this sound in this way, the abdomen withdraws and the huiyin cavity is held up. This is the key to store your qi and jing. The second way of making the heng sound is considered partially yang with some yin. It is made while exhaling with the mouth closed and it is used when you are interested in exerting jing but still wish to retain some of the power you are manifesting. The abdomen will be pushed out and the huiyin cavity will also be pushed out. To practice these two methods of producing heng, stand in the ma bu stance with your hands placed over your lower dan tian area. Next, inhale abruptly then allow the exhalation to relax out of the body. For each inhale draw in the abdomen and huiyin cavity while simultaneously making the heng sound. It is not a loud gasp but a soft heng sound that you will hear when you draw the air deep into the lungs. When exhaling, allow the abdomen and huiyin cavity to relax outward. You may practice this for a few minutes; however, if you feel you are becoming lightheaded you should relax and return to normal breathing. The second way of practicing the heng sound is also done while standing in the ma bu position with the hands placed on the lower dan tian. While inhaling, you will gently withdraw your abdomen and huiyin cavity. Then, exhaling, expand the abdomen and huiyin cavity with a more concentrated effort. Keep your mouth closed and express the heng sound. This should also be done for a few minutes.

The other sound is the ha (哈) sound. It is a pure yang sound and it is made when exhaling, and the abdomen and huiyin cavity are pushed out. This sound assists in the manifestation of the action as well as raises the spirit during the manifestation of jing.

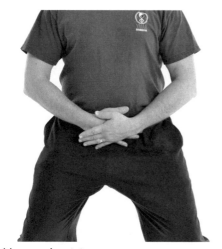
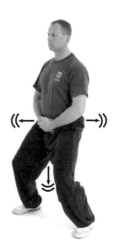

Ha sound training.

To train the ha sound, stand in the ma bu stance with your right hand placed on your dan tian. Place your left hand over the right hand. Inhale slowly and deeply while withdrawing your abdomen and rolling the hands into the lower dan tian area. Exhale and open your mouth while sounding out a long ha sound. At this point you are not forcefully shouting the sound. It should be a whispering ha sound. The hands will also roll outward with the abdomen expanding on the exhalation. Perform this action for a few repetitions until you are comfortable with the action.

Next, make the sound more pronounced. Resume the ma bu stance with your hands placed on the lower dan tian, Inhale slowly and deeply once again while rolling your hands over the dan tian area and withdrawing the abdomen. Exhale forcefully with your abdomen expanding, hands rolling outward, and a short but loud ha sound. Practice this exercise for a few repetitions. Please note: if at any time you become even slightly nauseous you should immediately stop this exercise and return to normal abdominal breathing to calm the body down.

Tips to Avoid Common Errors. The most common error is making the sound in your throat area. You may feel an irritation of the larynx and find your throat getting sore. To avoid such an irritation, you need to be sure the sound is expressed more from the exhalation through your diaphragm. Additionally, you need to allow the sound to escape out your mouth and be careful not to tense your neck and the surrounding area too much. Doing so will trap your qi and begin to cause a headache.

2.5 Martial Grand Qi Circulation

Grand qi circulation (da zhou tian, 大周天) is an advanced qigong qi circulation practice that conditions the twelve primary qi channels and two major vessels. This training involves self-cultivation (circulation within your own body), mutual cultivation with partners, and mutual cultivation with nature.

Martial grand qi circulation is another form of grand qi circulation. As it implies, it focuses on utilizing the grand qi circulation for martial purposes. The concern of martial artists is to build up this qi level to enhance their defensive and offensive skills. For defense the martial artists' the goal is to build qi and circulate it efficiently to the skin and beyond. The intent is to increase the sensitivity of the skin to be able to improve their listening, connecting, adhering, and following jing. The more skilled you are at sensing an opponent's intent, the better you will be able at neutralizing your opponent. It is said that when your qi can be transported strongly to your skin, it will cover your body like a cloud of energy. The stronger your qi, the thicker the cloud will be.

Offensively speaking, a martial artist needs to increase qi levels and circulate it efficiently to support the effectiveness of their striking. For taijiquan practitioners, their goal is to be able to effectively strike cavities. The highest level of taijiquan application is having an overabundant amount of qi such that touching an opponent results in qi being transported through the opponent's cavities.

In this section and in this book we will introduce exercises related to the self-cultivation and mutual cultivation with a partner. It is crucial that you already have knowledge of and have practiced both normal abdominal and reverse abdominal breathing as well as small circulation. You also should have some knowledge of two-gate and four-gate breathing techniques before attempting to practice martial grand circulation. Without practicing the techniques of building qi and learning how to circulate it, you will not reach a deeper level of training. We will highlight these techniques briefly here. However, we highly recommend you refer to other sources of information if you wish to increase your knowledge of this subject. Sources of this type of training may be found at YMAA Publication Center.

1. Yongquan Breathing (Yongquan Xi, 湧泉息)

In yongquan breathing, in coordination with real dan tian breathing, (you) use the yi to lead the qi from the real dan tian to the yongquan cavity. There it communicates with external qi. External qi enters through the yongquan cavity and the yi leads it back to the real dan tian. This is what Zhuang Zi called "sole breathing." Zhuang Zi said: "Normal people's breathing uses the throat while truthful persons' breathing uses the sole." Truthful persons imply those Dao searchers who have trained the qi and have reached a profound stage of (spiritual) purity and truth. In order to practice yongquan breathing, (you) must first understand the keys of embryonic breathing. Under the condition of soft and slender breathing, use the yi to lead the qi to the soles and then return it back (to the real dan tian). Han Xu Zu said: "What is sole breathing? It means continuous without broken, soft and slender as it is existing." From this, (you) can see that, with the prior condition of a profound level of regulating the breathing, yi is the foundation of success in yongquan breathing. When yi is strong, the qi is sufficient and when yi is weak, the qi is deficient.

湧泉息者，即是在配合真丹田呼吸下，以意引氣由真丹田至湧泉穴與外氣相通，再由湧泉穴由外納氣意引歸返真丹田之謂也。此亦即莊子所謂之踵息矣。莊子曰：〝常人之息以喉，真人之息以踵。〞真人者，尋道撲實練氣至深之人。為求湧泉之息，必先懂胎息之竅，在綿綿呼吸中，以意引氣來回足踵也者。涵虛祖曰：〝踵也者，相接不斷，綿綿若存也。〞由此可知，在深度的調息前題下，意為湧泉息之本。意強，氣厚，意弱，氣薄。

The yongquan (K-1) (湧泉) (i.e., gushing spring) cavities belong to the kidney primary channel and are located on the bottom of the feet. These two cavities are two major gates that are beneficial in maintaining health through the regulation the body's qi. They are also used for rooting conditioning. In taijiquan and pushing hands training you need to have a strong foundation, or root, to exert jing and to neutralize incoming forces into emptiness. It requires you to be able to lead your qi through your feet. Being able to do this also requires that you maintain a high level of sensitivity with these cavities. Success, of course, depends on how strong and concentrated your

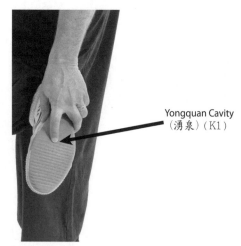

Yongquan Cavity
(湧泉) (K1)

Location of yongquan cavity.

mind (yi, 意) is. The stronger you can focus your qi to the area needed, the stronger the qi will flow. However, even when the yi is strong, the breathing must be soft and slender so the qi's flow can be smooth and continuous.

When you practice yongquan breathing, you may either lie down or stand up. Standing yongquan breathing is commonly used to establish a firm root in martial arts training. The main focus for this training is that your exhalation is longer than your inhalation. This means that first you inhale deeply and then you exhale slowly and finely while using your mind to lead the qi to the yongquan cavity and beyond. The key to establishing a strong yi is squatting down while imagining you are pushing your feet downward into the ground. When your exhalation is longer than your inhalation, it does not mean you release more carbon dioxide out and take in less oxygen. It

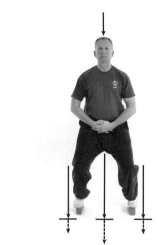

Standing yongquan training.

just means that the flow rates are different. When you exhale slower and longer, your mind is calmer and your concentration is stronger. Naturally, the flow rate of the exhalation is less than that of the inhalation.

Initial standing training will be done on the ground. As you begin to feel the qi flow deeper below your feet, you will begin to train while standing on bricks. If you can comfortably stand on top of two or three vertically stacked bricks while leading the qi through the bottom of the lowest bricks, your yi is considered to be strong and your flow of qi is considered deep. If you are able to reach this level your root will be at least three feet under your soles once you remove all of the bricks and stand on the ground.

2. Laogong Breathing (Loagong Xi, 勞宮息)

The laogong cavity (P-8) (勞宮) is located at the center of the palms and it belongs to the pericardium primary qi channel (xin bao luo jing, 心包絡經). These cavities are also major gates and they assist in the regulation of qi in the body. Laogong breathing increases the sensitivity of the palms for listening, adhering, and following skills. Additionally, you will learn to lead qi through these cavities for manifesting jing when you counterattack your opponents. To practice this type of training, stand in the ma bu stance with your hands at waist level and your palms facing downward. Focus on exhaling longer than inhaling just as you did in the yongquan breathing section.

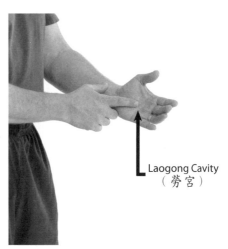

Laogong Cavity
(勞宮)

Location of laogong cavity.

Use your yi to focus leading the qi through your laogong cavities. To assist in leading qi through this area it is recommended to slightly move the palms downward while exhaling. You may also use the image of crushing a giant beach ball into the ground to increase the intensity. Over time you will sense the qi traveling through this area more easily and need less physical movement to assist you in leading your qi.

For your initial training remain stationary with your hands in front of your body. As you are able to perform this exercise with more ease you will adapt this feeling into the movements of taiji pushing hands.

3. Four Gates Breathing (Si Xin Xi, 四心息)

In pushing hands training one must be able to lead incoming forces into emptiness and manifest jing all while maintaining a firm root and balanced body. This is known as "central equilibrium" (zhong ding, 中定). It is written, " If there is a top, there is a bottom; if there is a front, there is a back; if there is a left, there is a right."[8] From this statement master Zhang, San-Feng (張三豐) discusses the importance of maintaining your central equilibrium. Through training you will be able to keep your center to a point and be able to readjust yourself to maintain this point. The location of this point is your real dan tian or your physical center of gravity. Using four gates breathing will allow you to focus on the location of this point and be able to manifest jing while maintaining your root. Additionally, you will be able to keep your center while others attempt to find it and uproot you.

Four gates breathing follows the practicing methods of laogong and yongquan breathing. If you practice this lying down do not cross your legs. When the legs are in the crossed position, qi flow stagnates in the kua (waist) area, defeating the intent of your training. Whether you're standing or lying down, inhale while leading your qi to the real dan tian area then slowly exhale while your mind (yi) leads your qi along the legs and arms and out their respective cavities. Over time you will feel all four of your cavities breathing with you.

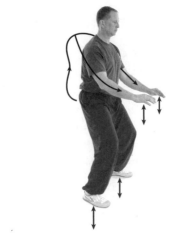

Four gates breathing.

4. Five Gates Breathing (Wu Xin Xi, 五心息)

The next stage of training is five gates breathing. The fifth gate is the baihui (Gv-20) (百會) cavity located on the top of the head. It is associated with the governing vessel and is considered the residence of the spirit (shen, 神). It is also paired with and lies vertically opposite the huiyin cavity. Fifth gate breathing may also be referred to as the martial side of spiritual breathing (shen xi, 神息). You are using this technique to raise up the spirit so the other four gates reach their maximum.

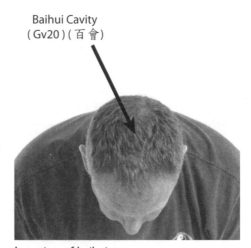

Baihui Cavity (Gv20) (百會)

Location of baihui.

Five gates breathing means that, after (you have) regulated the four gates breathing to the point that regulating is unnecessary, then (you) add the fifth gate's breathing. The first possible fifth gate is the baihui. The baihui cavity connects to the huiyin through the chong mai (i.e., thrusting vessel). The chong mai is what is called the spinal cord and is a highly electrically conductive material. Therefore, though the baihui and the huiyin are located in two different places, their functions are connected and act as one. The huiyin is the most yin place in the entire body, while the baihui is the residence of the yang-shen (i.e., yang spirit) and is the most yang place in the entire body. The huiyin is the yin meeting place of the four yin vessels—conception, thrusting, yin heel, and yin linking vessels and is the key controlling gate of the entire body's yin and yang. To qi practitioners, it is the secret gate for leading qi. When the huiyin is held upward, the huiyin gate is closed and the body's qi is condensed inward into the bone marrow, the spirit is converged and the qi is gathered, the entire body turns yin, and consequently, the jing is stored. Conversely, when the huiyin is pushed out, the huiyin gate is opened, qi is released from the four yin vessels, the yang spirit is raised up, the entire body turns yang, and consequently, the jing is emitted. One store and one emit, this is the key cycle of the internal jing's storing and emitting.[9]

五心息者，在四心息調至不調而自調之境地時，即加添第五心之息。
第五心者，百會也。百會由衝脈相通於會陰。衝脈者，脊髓神經也，
特高之電導體也。因而百會與會陰雖於上下兩處，其作用唯一己矣。
會陰為陰為全身最陰之所，百會為陽為陽神顯陽之地，亦是全身最陽
之處。會陰者，四陰脈，任、衝、陰蹻、陰維脈交會之所，是全身陰
陽控制之關，是練氣者引氣之竅門。會陰上提，會陰鎖，氣內斂入骨
髓，神凝氣聚，全身趨陰，勁由之而蓄。反之，會陰下推，會陰開，
氣由四陰脈外放，陽神上提，全身趨陽，勁由之而發。一蓄一發，此
為內勁蓄發關要之鑰。

Fifth gate breathing is the most important key to the jing's manifestation. The reason behind this is the relationship of the yi and qi within the five gates. Using five gates breathing training, the yi and the qi of this fifth gate are balanced with the other four gates. When the yi and qi are strong in this gate, the yi and qi of the other four gates will also be strong, and the jing's manifestation will be powerful.

The baihui is the residence of the spirit (shen, 神), as mentioned above, and the huiyin (Co-1) (會陰) is the storage place of water. The shen is yang while water is yin. That is why the shen is commonly called yang shen (陽神) while the huiyin (Co-1) (會陰) is called sea bottom (haidi, 海底). The huiyin is the place that connects the real dan tian and the four yin vessels and thus stores the qi, while the shen is the place that governs the effectiveness of the qi's manifestation. In fact, these two cavities are the two poles of the body's central energy that runs through the spinal cord. When this central energy is strong, the body's vital force is strong. Naturally, the jing manifested will be powerful and precise.

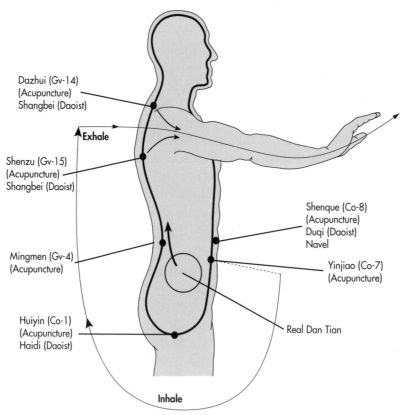

Dazhui (Gv-14)
(Acupuncture)
Shangbei (Daoist)

Exhale

Shenzu (Gv-15)
(Acupuncture)
Shangbei (Daoist)

Shenque (Co-8)
(Acupuncture)
Duqi (Daoist)
Navel

Mingmen (Gv-4)
(Acupuncture)

Yinjiao (Co-7)
(Acupuncture)

Huiyin (Co-1)
(Acupuncture)
Haidi (Daoist)

Real Dan Tian

Inhale

Location of the Yinjiao and Mingmen cavities in Grand Transportation Gong,

According to Chinese medicine, huiyin means "yin meeting" and is the gate that controls the qi's storage or release from the four yin vessels. When the huiyin is pushing out, the qi in the four yin vessels is released, and when this cavity is held upward, the qi is preserved. This implies that when you store your jing, you are holding this cavity upward while inhaling and when you emit your jing, you are pushing this cavity outward while exhaling.

(Throughout your) entire body, your mind is on the spirit of vitality (jing shen), not on the qi. (If concentrated) on the qi, then stagnant. This is the fifth gate breathing. Spirit (i.e., shen) is the master of the qi's circulation. When the spirit is high, the qi's circulation is natural, strong, and smooth. When the spirit is low, then the qi is stagnant, weak, and hard to circulate. This is the secret key to jing manifestation.

武禹襄云；〝全身意在精神，不在氣，在氣則滯。〞此即意第五心之呼吸也。神為氣行之主宰，神高，氣行自然沛而順，神低，氣滯弱而難行。此為勁發之訣竅也。

In this passage Wǔ, Yu-Xiang (武禹襄) discusses one's focus on the spirit and not the qi itself. If you focus on the qi itself you are not leading it but rather keeping it stagnant. Keeping a focused effort on raising the spirit to higher levels leads to a stronger, more effective qi flow. The key to leading your qi efficiently is to develop a sense of having an enemy. This means that you have an imaginary opponent. When your mind is on your opponent, your yi will lead the qi there for jing manifestation. The strength of your qi depends on the strength of your yi. However, the strength of your yi depends on your fighting spirit and morale. When this spirit is high, your alertness and awareness will also be high. Naturally, the qi can then be directed efficiently.

5. Grand Transportation Gong (Zhou Tian Mai Yun Gong, 周天邁運功)

Grand transportation gong is one of the main internal training exercises that can assist a taijiquan practitioner to enhance the circulation of qi to the arms so that martial power (i.e., jing, 勁) can be manifested to a higher level. In this training, qi is lead up the spine and out the arms through the laogong cavities along with an additional flow of qi that is led into the spine through the mingmen (命門) (Gv-4) cavity. Qi is also led downward through the legs in order to balance this qi led upward.

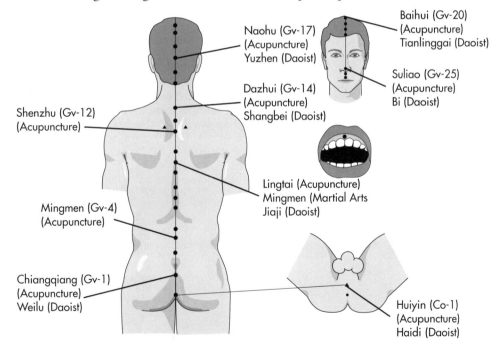

Theoretically there are two gates that connect to the lower dan tian. One is located on the front of the body and is known as the yinjiao (Co-7, 陰交) cavity. The other is located between the L2 and L3 vertebrae on your back. It is called the mingmen (Gv-4, 命門) cavity. Chinese martial artists discovered that if they were able to lead additional qi out through this cavity it would enhance their martial power. This is one of the paths in self-internal grand circulation. Taijiquan ancestor Wǔ, Yu-Xiang (武禹襄) said: "Power is emitted from the spine." (力由脊發) also, "(The mind) leads the qi flowing back and forth, adhering to the back, then condensing into the spine."[10] All of this implies that leading the qi upward through the spine is a way of storing the jing. Using this method of leading your qi is a key to jing manifestation.

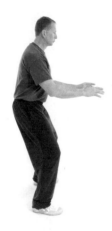

Step into your ma bu stance and place your hands, palms facing down, in front of your lower dan tian area.

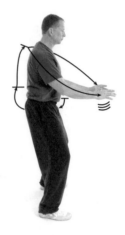

Inhale and begin to wave your spine while leading qi from your dan tian, out the yinjiao (Co-7) (陰交) cavity, past the huiyin (Co-1) (會陰) cavity, and up past the ming-men (Gv-4) (命門) cavity.

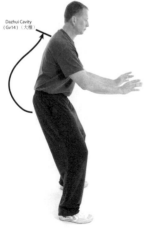

Continue to wave your spine while leading the qi up the spine to the dazhui (Gv-14) (大椎) cavity.

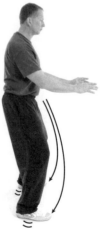

Qi is also led down the legs to balance qi led upward.

Step into your ma bu stance and place your hands, palms facing down, in front of your lower dan tian area. Inhale and begin to wave your spine while leading qi from your dan tian, out the yinjiao (Co-7) (陰交) cavity, past the huiyin (Co-1) (會陰) cavity, and up past the mingmen (Gv-4) (命門) cavity. Passing the mingmen (Gv-4) (命門) cavity, continue to inhale and vertically wave the spine. This will help open the mingmen (Gv-4) (命門) cavity and allow more qi to pass out of this cavity from the dan tian area. Continue to wave your spine while leading the qi up the spine to the dazhui (Gv-14) (大椎) cavity. From this position begin to exhale while leading the qi out through the arms. The waving action of the spine is carried out through the shoulders, the elbows, and ends out in your hands. Your hands will perform the push (an, 按), or settle the wrist movement as the qi is led out beyond them. Additionally, lead qi downward from the real lower dan tian area through the bottom of your feet. This entire movement should be practiced at a slow pace until the action becomes natural throughout the body. Your hands should remain at waist height initially, then you will vary the height of your hands up to shoulder height. As the action becomes more comfortable, increase the speed of the movement. With the increase in speed, the action becomes more of a whipping action where you will find your hands will snap back toward the body. You may also add the ha sound to assist in manifestation of the action as well. Practice this exercise until you are comfortable performing it. The movements and breathing should be natural and unified.

6. Skin-Marrow Breathing (Fu Sui Xi, 膚髓息)

Skin breathing is also referred to as body breathing (ti xi, 體息). In addition to opening the twelve primary channels and two main vessels, a taiji pushing hands practitioner must learn to open all the channels of the body. There are thousands of small qi branches, or luo (絡), that branch out from the main channels to the skin and into every part of the body. Among the benefits of opening these channels with an abundant flow of qi is the increased sensitivity of the skin. For the taiji pushing hands practitioner this means increased awareness of the opponent's actions. The ability to listen, attach, adhere, and follow incoming forces becomes second nature. Over time you will see the intent prior to the movement. It has been written that in taijiquan you do not move if your opponent doesn't move. When they move you are already there. This implies that when you are able to build qi to its highest levels and are able to circulate this qi strongly throughout the body and mind you will be able to sense your opponent's intentions. If they don't move you do not move. If they begin to attack you will be able to sense it and react first.

In order to practice this method of breathing you need to learn to open as many of the luo cavities as possible. You need to build qi up to the point that it overflows from open cavities into others. You need to continuously train your dan tian, filling it with qi and causing it to vibrate like a drum. You then need to extend it out beyond your skin. There are multiple methods of training this such as taiji coiling exercises, sitting meditation, or even simply walking down the street. To train, imagine your lower dan tian area is a sphere. As you exhale, imagine the sphere expands out beyond your body. This imagery expands your qi outward as well. You may also use this method when training any of the other exercises here in the book.

2.6 Taiji Ball Qigong

Taiji ball qigong training is a qigong exercise practice that uses balls of various sizes and materials to train the mind and body to higher levels of conditioning for both health and martial arts. It was derived from Da Mo's muscle/tendon changing and marrow/brain washing qigong (yi jin jing/xi sui jing, 易筋經 / 洗髓經). Muscle/tendon changing is used to condition the physical body from weak to strong so the jing manifested can be powerful and effective. Marrow/brain washing trains a practitioner in how to use the mind to lead the qi to circulate through the entire body more efficiently. In addition, this training also focuses on how to store the qi in the bone marrow and to lead the qi upward through the thrusting vessel (i.e., chong mai, 衝脈) to the brain to raise up the spirit of vitality (jing shen, 精神). When the spirit is raised, the fighting morale will be high and the entire body can be a powerful and effective fighting unit. This qigong was commonly practiced in ancient times when martial arts played an important role in society.

Traditionally, taiji ball qigong training was a very important training for many external and internal styles. The reason it is so effective is because taiji ball qigong, using wood (internal styles) or rock (external styles) balls in the hands, helps focus the training in round movements. Consequently, this training is able to increase the endurance, strength, mobility, and flexibility of the practitioner's physical body, especially the torso. Not only that, taiji ball qigong trains a practitioner in how to use their mind to lead the qi more efficiently so the power can be manifested to its maximum strength. Two-person exercises allow the practitioner to increase their sensitivity to an opposing force and enhance the ability to neutralize the force. The trainings used to practice the patterns were usually created following a style's specialties and techniques.

Due to their effectiveness and efficiency in training a student to become a proficient fighter, the training methods were usually kept secret. It was also because of this secrecy that the training has almost become lost today. Now, only a few old masters actually know it.

In taijiquan, training taiji ball qigong can offer you the following benefits:

Physical

1. Train roundness of the movements and feeling. Roundness is a crucial key of coiling and neutralization in taijiquan and pushing hands training.

2. Strengthen torso, especially lower back and chest.

3. Recondition ligaments and tendons (i.e., joints).

4. Loosening the hips and waist, keys of pushing hands.

5. Move the entire body as one unit with firm root and balance.

6. Establish a firm root and balance during stepping.

7. Train endurance, the crucial key to surviving in a long battle.

Mental

1. Protect and feel center and balance.

2. Learn to use the mind to lead the qi (martial grand circulation).

3. Train focus, alertness, and awareness.

4. Familiar with round feeling and movements.

5. Practice the feeling of attachment, listening, stick, and adhere, which are crucial key skills of taiji pushing hands.

As you can see there are many benefits of taiji ball qigong training. Taiji ball qigong is probably one of the most effective and efficient qigong practices for both martial arts and health. It emphasizes not just physical but also mental training. If you are interested in taiji ball qigong, please refer to our book and DVD *Tai Chi Ball Qigong*, which can be found at YMAA Publication Center.

In the following section we will first introduce you to a few theories pertaining to taiji ball exercises. Next we will demonstrate a few exercises that can be used for enhancing taiji pushing hands training. Keep in mind, to properly train taiji ball, it is highly recommended you begin your training with the solo exercises of circling, rotating, and wrap-coiling before attempting to train the advanced levels of exercises.

The training of this gong (i.e., gongfu) can be divided into three levels. The first level is taiji ball practice without a ball. The training of this level aims for the smoothness of the basic movements, using the yi to lead the qi, and also the harmonization and coordination of the internal ball and external ball. The internal ball is hidden internally at the real dan tian which belongs to yin, while the external ball is manifested externally between the palms and belongs to yang. From the internal ball's rotating and circular movements, the patterns are delivered to the external ball through the spine. At the beginning, the movements are slow so the effect of using the yi to lead the qi can be achieved. When the movements are slow, the feeling can be deep. This means the gongfu of internal vision (i.e., feeling) can also be deep. When the feeling is deep, the yi can also reach deeply. In this case, the state of leading the qi to "no place cannot be reached" can be achieved.[11]

此功之練法可分三段。其初段為無球之太極球練習。此段之練習在求
基本動作之順利，以意引氣，內球與外球輾轉之調合諧和。內球在真
丹田藏於內為陰，外球在手掌間顯於外為陽。由內球氣之動與動作之
輾轉，由脊椎遞送而至外球。初行時，動作緩慢以求以意引氣之效。
動作慢，感覺深，亦即內視功夫深也。當然，感覺深，意亦可深，而
氣可引至無所不到之境界。

There are three levels of taiji ball training: training without a ball, training with a ball and, again, training without a ball. The first level of training focuses on the physical movements of the spine and body and the imaginary ball. You also begin to feel a secondary ball located within the lower dan tian. Movement is initiated from this internal ball, follows the path up through the spine, and is externally manifested between the palms. While you are doing this, not only can the movements be directed by the waist, the qi can also be led through grand circulation from the real dan tian smoothly to the palms.

At the beginning of the training, the movements should be slow, which allows your yi to reach a deeper level of activating body movement. In addition, this will help you use your mind to lead the qi through grand circulation. If your yi can reach to the skin and beyond (i.e., guardian qi) (wei qi, 衛氣) as well as to the marrow (i.e., marrow qi) (sui qi, 髓氣), then you will be able to store the qi using the bone marrow and also manifest it externally to the skin surface for power manifestation.

After practicing to proficiency in the first level, so that the twelve basic movements can be as smooth as you wish, you can then hold a taiji ball and again train the twelve basic movements. Generally, a taiji ball can be made from wood or stone. Those who emphasize training li (i.e., muscular power) usually use a stone ball while those who emphasize training qi usually use a wooden ball. Those who practice taijiquan like to use a wooden ball simply because it can be used to train qi. At the beginning, use a ball that is smaller, lighter, and less dense. After the muscles/tendons and bones have become stronger, then use a ball that is heavier, larger, and denser. Also at the beginning, due to the weight of the ball, the muscles are more tensed and consequently the qi is hard to circulate. However, after practicing for a period of time, the body becomes stronger and this will allow (you) to be more relaxed. Only then (you) will advance further and use (your) mind to lead the qi following the fibers of the wooden ball to communicate between the palms. This can gradually change to go against the fibers and again use the yi to lead the qi to communicate between the palms.

在初段功練到一個程度之後，十二基本動作得心應手後，則手握太極球再依十二基本式練習。普通之太極球可木製或石製。練力者，多用石製，練氣者，多用木製。練太極拳者，喜用木製球練氣。初用質鬆、較輕、較小之球。在筋骨較強後，可用質硬、較重、較大之球。初練時，因球沈重，肌肉繃緊，氣因而難行。練到一段時間後，身強體壯，身體輕鬆。此時進一步用意先依質紋而引氣過球，漸而用意逆紋而引氣過球，以達高層次。

Once you have become proficient in the twelve basic movements of taiji ball training you will begin training with a ball. External styles, which focus on the strength of the muscles and tendons at the beginning, usually use a stone ball for this training. However, internal stylists favor a ball made from wood, which allows them to lead the qi through the ball more easily and smoothly.

Training at this level will cause a temporary stagnation to the flow of qi. This is due to the physical weight of the ball being added to the body that in turn will cause you to be somewhat tense. Over time your body will adapt and the tension will disappear. Qi will once again flow smoothly.

Initially, you will train with the grain of the wood being perpendicular to your hands. This will assist in the flow of qi from hand to hand. When you are able to pass qi easily through the ball you will change the direction of the grain to face parallel to the hands. If you are still able to communicate the qi between both palms, you have reached a profound level of taiji ball qigong.

The last level of practice is returning to the stage of practice without a ball. At this time, because there is no wood, the body can reach to its extreme state of relaxation and softness, the yi can reach its peak, and the qi can be lead as you wish without stagnation. In this case, the achievement for both internal and external goals have been accomplished. When using (these skills) to push hands or encounter an opponent, there is more than enough capability to handle the job.

最後段之練習，回到無球之練習。此時，因無木球，身體可鬆軟至極點。意可達高峰，氣之行隨心所欲。如此內外兼修，用之於推手應敵，綽綽有餘。

The final stage of taiji ball training is repeating the twelve patterns without a ball. Your body will be able to reach its maximum relaxation and softness, your mind will be strong, and you will be able to lead the qi strongly and effectively.

After you have completed these twelve basic patterns of taiji ball training, you should mix them any way you like and turn these twelve dead patterns into a living one. Imagine you are pushing hands with someone and apply all of the taiji ball movements in the actions. In doing so, you will have made taiji ball training creative and alive.

2.6.1 Self Practice

In the following section we will describe a few exercises related to adhering to the ball while it is on a table. The purpose of this training is to continue to increase your listening and adhering skills beyond the ball. Again, these exercises are just a few taken from a collection of exercises you should practice when engaging in taiji ball training.

Adhering to the Ball

1. Wrap Coiling on the Table (Zhuo Shang Zhan Zhuan, 桌上輾轉)

The following exercise is used to enhance the skills of adhering to an object while leading it around the table. It will also train the joints of your hips, knees, and ankles as you twist your body back and forth throughout the circling of the ball. Finally you will learn to connect the lower body with the upper body and to lead your force from the ground through the spine and out through your hands.

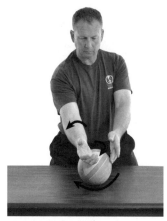 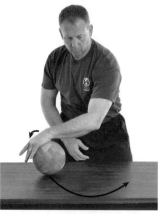 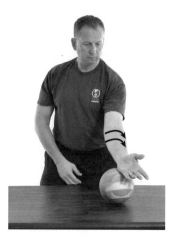

Wrap coiling training: right hand.
Wrap coiling training: left hand.

To begin, slightly squat into your ma bu stance in front of a table with the ball on the table. Starting with your right hand on the ball, palm down; you will begin to inhale while circling the ball toward you in a clockwise path on the table. Continue to circle the ball to your left and then forward while exhaling. Move your hand so that the ball rolls around the side of the fingers and then to the backside of your palm. This is the wrap coiling action of the hand on the ball. As the ball continues on its path across the table and passes your centerline, rotate your hand so the palm rests on the ball again. Continue to circle the ball clockwise back to the original starting position and repeat the previous steps while moving the ball in a clockwise manner over the table. Generally speaking, close your chest as the ball moves toward your body and open the chest as it moves away from the body. With respect to your breathing, inhale as the ball moves toward you and exhale as it moves away from your body. Please note that you are not confined to using your hand. As you become more comfortable with this action you can use your wrist and forearm to circle the ball accordingly. You can change the size of the circling to a point where the ball remains relatively in front of your body on the table. Your hand performs the wrap coiling action around the ball while it circles in place. Continue to practice this exercise until the ball moves in the clockwise circle smoothly and uninterrupted, then practice the same exercise using your left hand. In this case the ball will move in a counterclockwise direction. Next, learn to change the direction of the movement using what is called the yin-yang exchange. Here you will use the center section of the yin-yang symbol to change direction of the circling This action prevents you from stopping the movement in order to change directions. To practice this, wrap coil the ball in the clockwise direction and pick a point of the circle where you can move the ball into the center and out the opposite side. Reaching the

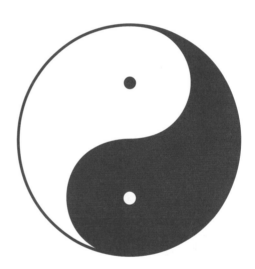

Yin Yang Symbol

other side, you will begin to wrap coil the ball in the opposite direction with the same hand. Continue to circle the ball counterclockwise while wrap coiling the right hand in the counterclockwise motion as well. Do this until you can do it comfortably and smoothly then begin to exchange wrap coiling clockwise and counterclockwise using the right hand. You should be able to change directions as well as the size of the wrap coiling smoothly and continuously.

Once you are able to perform this action, repeat the exercise for your left hand. Your left hand begins to perform its wrap coiling in a counterclockwise direction, and the ball travels in a counterclockwise motion around the table. Once again you can change the size of the wrap coiling pattern as well as change the direction of the ball using the yin-yang symbol exchanging. The goal is to be able to perform this smoothly and uninterruptedly. You should be able to exchange anywhere in the circling action.

Finally, move to the last set of exercises where you change back and forth between hands while circling the ball around the table. The main concept is to be able to change hands and direction of circling without stopping the motion of the ball. This freestyle action will move continuously throughout. Pushing hands practitioners must be able to redirect incoming forces without using force to stop the action and change direction. This exercise will assist you in accomplishing this task by teaching you to control the direction of the ball through adhering to it and being able to change directions as well as hands without stopping the movement of the ball.

To illustrate this exercise, begin with the right hand wrap coiling while moving the ball in a clockwise direction on the table just as you did in the previous exercise. To make the exchange to the opposite hand, simply follow the clockwise direction of the ball and place the left hand on the ball while removing the right hand. From this position continue to circle the ball in this direction unless you wish to perform a yin-yang exchange. You should continue to practice exchanging directions and hands until you are able to do so continuously and smoothly without stopping the movement of the ball. Eventually you will also practice this with your eyes closed.

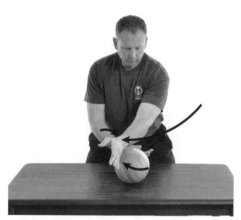

Wrap coiling training: changing hands.

Tips to Avoid Common Errors. A common error related to these exercises is not turning the waist while circling the ball on the table. Remember, the waist directs where the action is applied. You need to turn your waist not only to circle the ball but to redirect energy when it is applied to yourself. Additionally, you need to move the ball by using your entire body not just your hands. Finally, remember to open and close the chest while the ball is moved away and returned to you in the circle. The wardoff (peng, 掤) action must become a natural action so that anytime an opponent applies a force toward you it naturally occurs.

2. Train with Partners (Yu Ban Tong Lian, 與伴同練)

In the next set of exercises you will practice the movements with a partner. In addition to practicing your connecting, adhering, and sticking jing skills, you will also learn to train your distancing or central door training. For the taijiquan pushing hands practitioner, stay in a state of central equilibrium while keeping your central and empty door protected when your opponent attacks. You also need to learn how to close this distance when you are attacking. This certainly holds true for martial aspects of the taijiquan practitioner. The following are just a few of the many exercises that can be practiced to enhance these skills.

2.6.2 Freestyle Yin-Yang Circling while Rocking and Stepping

For the following exercises you and your partner will each place both hands on the ball. It should be noted that you should be familiar with the yin and yang aspects of circling the ball in both the vertical and horizontal plane. These exercises are described more fully in the book *Tai Chi Ball Qigong* we coauthored. The book as well as DVDs on taiji ball training are offered through the YMAA Publication Center website.

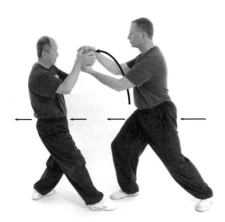

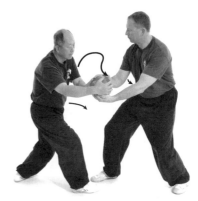

To begin, stand facing each other with your right legs forward. Place both hands on the ball. Move the ball toward your partner while rocking or shifting your weight forward. We are starting with the forward yang vertical circling here, but if you are familiar with these exercises you may begin in any direction.

As you shift forward, your partner shifts back and redirects the ball, circling it back toward you. In this example your partner circles the ball back toward you horizontally while shifting their weight forward. Again, you may choose any direction you wish and your opponent may do so as well.

Continue to rock back and forth, circling the ball in a freestyle manner until the ball flows smoothly throughout its path of circling. Once you are comfortable with this stage of the exercise, practice with stepping forward and backward.

For beginners, it is advisable to start by taking turns. Have one person step forward and backward for a period of time then have the opposite person step forward and backward. When you feel comfortable and you can smoothly execute the circling, either person may initiate the stepping.

In the next stage of this exercise, rock and step while using one hand on the ball.

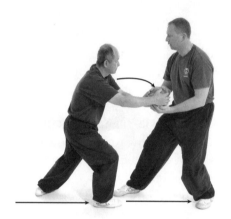

To step forward, begin from your most aft position with the ball. Turn the forward foot and begin to shift your weight forward while circling the ball in any direction. Slide the aft foot to the forward position as you continue to shift your weight and circle the ball. To step backward, begin from your most forward position. As you shift your weight back, slide the forward foot back while circling the ball in any direction.

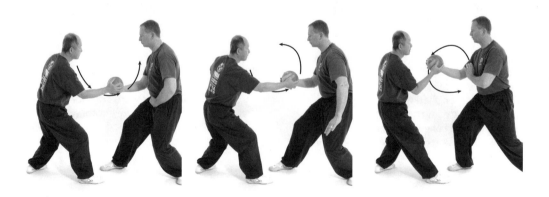

You and your partner each place one hand on the ball and place the other hand down by your lower dan tian. Then practice with the free hand out to your side, and finally by your shoulder.

Once you are able to perform this smoothly, practice exchanging to the opposite hand all while rocking and stepping.

Final stages of this exercise include being able to exchange hands while performing the freestyle circling technique, rocking and stepping while the eyes are closed and on bricks. Place the bricks strategically across the floor to allow you and your partner to step on them while you move across the area you are practicing. The order of brick training is to start with them flat on the ground (low), on the sides (middle), and then straight up and down (tall). Remember, training on bricks can be difficult. Be careful.

At this stage you are considered to be very proficient in sensitivity and rooting.

Tips to Avoid Common Errors. Common errors related to these exercises are not unlike those of the previous exercise. Beginners often forget to turn their waist to guide the ball to the left or right. Power manifestation must be initiated from the root of the foot. In addition, be careful not to lean and overextend yourself while practicing. This error will become more obvious when you practice on bricks. Another common error occurs with stepping. In the process of learning listening skills you and your partner may simultaneously step forward or backward and lose contact with the ball. Over time this should become less of a factor as you both build your listening skills.

1. Capture the Ball (Duo Qiu, 奪球)

This exercise is known as capturing the ball. In both taijiquan pushing hands and taijiquan martial applications, a person needs to learn how to give up force and flow with the opponent's energy, redirect the energy, then counterattack. In this exercise you are learning how not to use force to take a ball away from your opponent. This can be performed when moving forward or backward. In order to practice this exercise effectively, you will need to know how to rotate and wrap coil the taiji ball. These exercises are more fully explained in our book *Tai Chi Ball Qigong* and the accompanying DVDs.

For beginners, take turns capturing the ball. When you feel comfortable and can do it smoothly, freestyle back and forth.

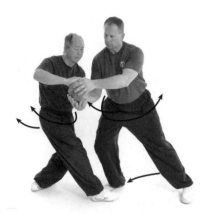 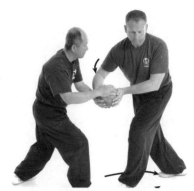

Stand facing your partner with your right legs forward and with both hands on the ball. Begin to rotate the ball in a freestyle manner while rocking. To capture the ball, start with rocking forward and rotating the ball such that the opponent begins to detach from the ball. Follow through by stepping forward and capturing the ball in your hands. Practice this a few times until it becomes smooth and effortless.

Next, practice capturing the ball while stepping backward. To perform this action, face your partner with right legs forward. Begin to rotate the ball while rocking back and forth just as you did in the previous exercise. To capture the ball, step back while rotating the ball. Once again practice this exercise until it becomes effortless to capture the ball from your partner. It should be captured without using a lot of force.

After you become comfortable with this part of the exercise, allow your partner to practice both the forward and backward capturing of the ball. Next, you and your partner will attempt to capture the ball in a nonsequential freestyle manner. Finally, you will both practice this with eyes closed.

Tips to Avoid Common Errors. The first and most obvious error in this exercise would be capturing the ball with force. This is completely opposite of what you are trying to accomplish here. The skill requires the development of listening jing to redirect the force and capture the ball.

2.7 Taiji Yin-Yang Symbol Sticking Hands Training

Traditionally, there are two taijiquan practices that a master would keep as top secrets until the students could be trusted. The reason these secrets were held was because these two practices are the key training to lead a taijiquan practitioner to a proficient level of fighting capability. These two practices are taiji ball qigong (太極球氣功) and taiji yin-yang symbol sticking hands practice.

From the last section we have demonstrated the benefits of taiji ball training and the use of it for assisting you in pushing hands training. Taiji ball qigong focuses on forward and backward circular movements vertically and horizontally for offensive and defensive jings' manifestation. Now let us look at the benefits of training taiji yin-yang symbol training.

Taiji yin-yang symbol sticking hands practice is also known as chan si jing (纏絲勁) (i.e., silk reeling jing) practice in Chen-style taijiquan. The practice consists of basic training exercises of tracing the yin-yang symbol in various postures. It includes both yang yin-yang symbol and yin yin-yang symbol. Usually, a beginner will practice the yang side first and after they have mastered the movements and can react skillfully, they then practice the yin side. Once these two symbols are mastered, you can go on to freestyle exercises that mix both yin and yang symbols. When this happens, you will be able to change your maneuver from yin to yang and yang to yin without a problem. In addition, through this practice, you will be able to build up a higher level of adhering, listening, and adhering jings, which are the crucial keys of taijiquan pushing hands and fighting capability. This will be practiced while solo as well as with another training partner. From this training, a practitioner will be able to improve:

1. Rooting and centering of the body.
2. The roundness of the movements.
3. The ability to move the entire body as a single unit, connected and continuous, from the root to the fingers.
4. Using the mind to lead the qi when needed for action.
5. The skills of attaching, listening, sticking, and adhering.
6. The feeling of the qi exchange with a partner.
7. The sensitivity to the opponent's body language.
8. Stepping with a firm root and balance.
9. The foundation of yin-yang strategy exchange, the crucial key of taijiquan martial applications.

Yin-yang symbol training contains many levels of training and is considered to be an integral part of taijiquan and taiji pushing hands training. As mentioner earlier, Master Zhang, San-Feng (張三豐) wrote, "The root is at the feet, jing (movement) is generated from the legs, mastered (i.e., controlled) by the waist, and manifested (i.e., expressed) from the fingers. From the feet to the legs to the waist must be integrated, and one unified qi. When moving forward or backward, (you can) catch the opportunity and gain the superior position."

Master Wǔ, Cheng-Qing (武澄清) wrote, "Hands and feet mutually follow each other and integrate with the waist and legs. Lead (the coming force) into emptiness, (its application) is marvelous and splendid."[12]

These statements express the fundamental emphasis and importance of the waist as the director of energy essential in both taiji pushing hands and freestyle fighting. They also teach us the necessity of the unification of upper and lower bodies. These exercises in yin-yang symbol training will also assist you in developing the connection of using both the upper body and lower body as one tool. When used with a partner, this type of training will reinforce the necessary skills of attaching, connecting, listening, following, and adhering. Additionally, this will also set the basis for how much force is necessary for a person to exert on their opponent when applying the offensive push maneuver in the pushing hands section of training.

In the following sections we will list a few theories related to yin-yang symbol training, followed by the exercises of yin-yang symbol training that are necessary to enhance your skills in pushing hands training. We encourage you to pursue all aspects of yin-yang symbol training to broaden your knowledge and expand your skills of taiji pushing hands. If you are interested to know more about taijiquan yin-yang symbol sticking hands training, please refer to the video *Taiji Yin Yang Sticking Hands* by YMAA Publication Center.

Yin-yang taiji circle coiling practice is a fundamental training gong of taijiquan's pushing hands, jing's emitting and neutralization, and free sparring. Those who practice the martial aspects of taijiquan must know this training. (This training) is called "chan si jing" (i.e., silk reeling jing) in Chen style and is called "yin-yang taiji circle sticking hands" in Yang style. This is because the taiji circle can be classified as yin and yang, two different circles. The yang circle emphasizes offense, seal, advance, and circling clockwise. The yin circle emphasizes defense, neutralization, withdrawing, and circling counterclockwise.[13]

陰陽太極圈纏手練習，乃太極拳推手、勁之發化、與自由散手之基本功。習太極拳武學者必須知之。在陳氏太極拳稱之為纏絲勁，楊氏卻稱之為陰陽太極圈纏手也。其因為太極圈之練習分為陰、陽兩手。陽手主攻、主封、主進，以右旋為主。陰手主守、主化、主退，以左旋為主。

Yin-yang symbol training is a fundamental training exercise of taijiquan pushing hands training. This training has four goals: 1. to improve the communication of the mind and the waist so the mind can control the waist efficiently, 2. to keep the joints soft so the jing can be led from the waist to the extremities without stagnation, 3. to manifest the jing as a soft whip, and 4. to use the mind to lead the qi from the real dan tian to the extremities so the jing can be manifested with maximum efficiency. Additionally, one will begin to understand the nature of yin and yang movements along with how to effectively transition between the two.

Taijiquan is considered an internal martial art that manifests soft jing patterns that are rooted in the feet and directed by the waist. The yin-yang symbol training exercises assist the practitioner in learning how to exert this power correctly. Chen stylists also train these exercises. It is known as "chan si jing" (纏絲勁), which means "silk reeling jing." A similar training has also been used in Yang style and is called "yin-yang taiji circle coiling and spiraling training" (陰陽太極圈纏手練習) or "yin-yang taiji symbol sticking hands training" (陰陽太極圈粘手練習).

In the taiji symbol, clockwise is classified as yang, while counterclockwise is classified as yin. In the practice of the taiji circle, the hand moves following the symbol and circles, rotates, coils, and spirals. The motion is initiated from the bottom of the feet, is controlled from the waist, and is then manifested into the fingers. From the bottom of the feet to the fingers, every section of each joint follows the symbol and circles, rotates, coils, and spirals. This is to train the entire body to be threaded as a single qi (i.e., single unit). From the bottom of the feet to the fingers acts as a soft whip. From the circling, rotating, coiling, and spiraling in the taiji symbol, (we also) search for the root of the jing's emitting and neutralization through the entire body. Furthermore, from practice, (we are) aiming for the regulating uniformity of the breathing and the smoothness of the qi's circulation. From the last stage of bagua taiji stepping training, (we) learn how to comprehend, familiarize, and experience the secret keys to the five phases steppings.

太極圖者，右旋為陽，左旋為陰。太極圈之練法，手依圖而輾轉、纏繞而行。圈由腳底起，控制於腰，而形於手指。由腳底至手指，節節關節有圖輾轉纏繞之。此練習全身關節之貫串一氣，由腳底至手指如軟鞭然。亦由太極圈之輾轉纏中，去求全身勁發、化之根由。更從練習中，去調合呼吸之均勻和運氣之通順。不但如此，在最終雙人之八卦太極行步練習中，去瞭解、熟悉，體驗五行步伐之訣竅。

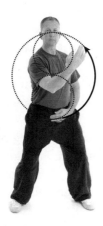

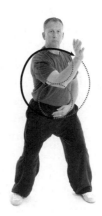

Right hand, taijiquan yang symbol direction.   Right hand, taijiquan yin symbol direction.

In yin-yang symbol training, the yin and yang aspects of the taiji symbols are classified as follows. When using your right hand, the yang side of the taiji symbol rotates clockwise and is mainly used for offense. The yin side of the taiji symbol rotates counterclockwise and is mainly used for defense. In the yang symbol, the jing is originated from the legs while the coiling is initiated from the center of the waist (i.e., real dan tian) and then gradually expands outward with circling, rotating, coiling, and spiraling motions until it reaches an imaginary opponent's body. From this training, a practitioner learns how to use the mind to lead the qi from the real dan tian to the extremities and also how to use the waist to direct the motion from the center to the target. In the yin symbol, again the jing is originated from the legs, the coiling is initiated from the opponent's body, and through circling, rotating, coiling, and spiraling motions, the circle is gradually reduced toward the center until it reaches the real dan tian. This symbol is used to neutralize and is mainly for defense.

There are many stages of taiji symbol training: from solo to matching, from stationary to moving, and from straight line to bagua circle stepping. Through rotation, the circle can be vertical, horizontal, large, and small. From this, you can see that the entire action is alive and variable. The final stage of two-person bagua circle stepping training is used to train the practitioner to step correctly with the taijiquan's five strategic stepping techniques that coordinate with the five phases (wuxing, 五行) (i.e., metal, wood, water, fire, and earth).

At the beginning of training, one hand moves following the pattern of the clockwise yang taiji symbol. First practice solo, follow the taiji symbol to circle and coil. After becoming familiar with the symbol pattern, (you) can enter two-person practice. Two-person practice can be classified as stationary, advance and retreat moving, advance and retreat parallel moving, and finally bagua taiji circle stepping practice. After (you have) mastered the movement of clockwise yang taiji symbol, then (you can) begin the practice of the counterclockwise yin taiji symbol. Its practice procedures are the same as those of yang taiji symbol, from solo to the two-person bagua taiji circle stepping. After (you) have practiced enough to reach a proficient level and all of the movements have become natural, then mix the clockwise and counterclockwise pattern in your practice. This will lead to the practice of freestyle yin-yang taiji symbols matching. In this stage, yin and yang, insubstantial and substantial strategies can be varied; sealing, emitting, neutralizing, and controlling as you wish. The opponent does not know you but you know the opponent.

初練時，手依右旋陽式太極圖之型為主而動。先由各人獨自練習，依太極圖輾轉而動。在熟悉圖型後，即可步入雙人練習。雙人練習，可分定步，前進與後退動步，前進與後退平行動步，最終為八卦太極行步之練習。在熟悉右旋陽式太極圖之動後，即可步入左旋陰式太極圖之動。練習程序與右旋陽式太極圖之練法同。由各人之練習，而終至雙人八卦太極行步之練習。在練到一切動作成自然後，右旋陽式與左旋陰式即混合著練，而成為自由陰陽太極圖對練。到此程度，陰陽、虛實由我變，封發化拿隨我意，敵不知我，我卻知敵。

Once you have mastered both yang and yin taiji symbol sticking hands training from solo until bagua taiji circle, then you begin to mix them up. Through these yin-yang interactions, hundreds of techniques are derived. In this case, yin and yang can be exchanged, and the insubstantial and substantial strategies are alive and controlled. When this happens, you will put your opponent into an urgent and disadvantageous situation and under your control. You will know your opponent but your opponent will not know you. From this, you can see that taiji symbol sticking hands training is the essence and the root of taijiquan fighting arts. That is the reason it has always been kept secret in the past.

2.7.1 Yang Symbol Training—Solo (Yang Quan Dan Lian, 陽圈單練)

1. Solo—Vertical (Dan Lian—Chui Zhi, 單練—垂直)

The first exercise is yang circling while in the stationary posture. Begin the practice with circling vertically using the right hand. A basic guide for practicing the yang symbol training is that the thumb will lead the hand throughout the yang circle. To further simplify the training process, the initial size of the vertical symbol will be described as follows. The lowest section will be approximately at the lower dan tian level. The highest point will be level with the eyes, or upper dan tian area. The width or sides of the symbol will be slightly wider than shoulder width. The center of the symbol will be heart or middle dan tian level. The waist will guide the hand throughout the

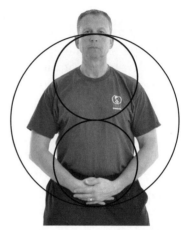

Perimeters for solo vertical yang symbol training.

symbol. In this beginning practice the symbol appears to be completely vertical. This is for training purposes. It is more of a sphere when performed correctly. In addition, you may change the size of the yin-yang symbol to any diameter once you are comfortable with the movements. Advanced levels of training will involve changing from vertical to horizontal, eventually leading to multiple spheres with no set size.

When applying the concepts of taiji yin and yang theory to this exercise, the palm of the hand is considered to be in a yin position when facing the body or the ground and in a yang position when facing away from the body or toward the sky. The direction of yang circling moves from center outward. When using the right hand, the yang direction is clockwise. When using the left hand, the yang direction is counterclockwise.

Stationary.

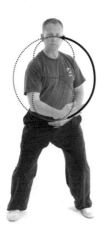

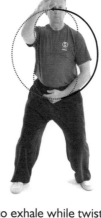

Stand in ma bu with the right hand placed in front of your body approximately at the lower dan tian height. With your chest closed, inhale deeply then begin to exhale while you twist your body to the left. With the thumb leading, the hand will start to circle forward and up along the outside section of the symbol.

Continue to exhale while twisting your body back to the right, opening the chest and leading the hand toward the top section of the symbol. On reaching the top of the symbol, rotate the palm down so the thumb may continue to lead in tracing the symbol.

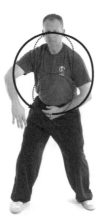

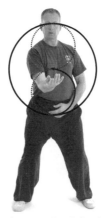

Begin to inhale while continuing to twist your body to the right and leading the hand back toward your body and down the opposite side of the symbol. Your hand will need to rotate slightly to allow the thumb to continue to lead the palm on the path of the symbol. Twist your body back to the left, close the chest once again, and lead your hand back to your original position facing forward. This completes the outside section of the symbol. Now, you pass through the center section.

This time twist your body back to the right while leading your hand through the center of the symbol while opening your chest and exhaling. Your hand will be heart level with your palm facing slightly toward the sky passing this point.

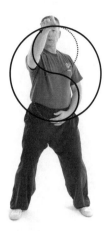

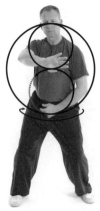

Twist your body back to the left while exhaling and continue to raise your hand up and away from your body as you did before. Continue to twist your body back to the right and raise your hand, rotating the palm so it begins to face the ground. Once again twist back to the left, ending with your chest open and your hand now eye level palm facing down.

Begin to inhale while you twist back to the right and draw your hand down toward your body. Initially you will trace the outside of the circle then move back into the center section. Continue to twist your body to the right while inhaling, closing your chest and drawing your hand down through the center of the symbol. You will pass once again through heart level.

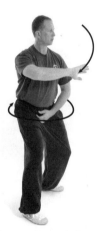

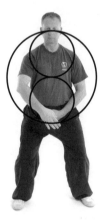

Pay attention to the area from the top to the heart level. Make sure your body is creating the action and the hand is drawn through the center of the symbol. If your body does not lead, there is an incorrect tendency to raise the elbow well above the wrist when tracing this part of the symbol.

To complete the symbol pattern, continue to twist your body to the right while closing the chest and drawing the hand down toward the lower right side of the symbol. Finally, twist back to the left, ending with the hand in front of the dan tian area, palm facing your body.

Repeat this exercise using your right hand until you are able to trace the pattern smoothly using the waist to direct your hand and opening and closing your chest at the appropriate times.

Once you are comfortable with training the right hand, practice with the left hand. The movements required to trace the symbol remain the same as they are with the right hand. The main difference is the left hand will perform the action by initially circling in a counterclockwise direction. Remember that the thumb leads the hand throughout the symbol. This should help you when trying to remember which way you need to turn. Due to the similarity, we will not describe this exercise in full detail. But repeat this exercise for the left hand until you are able to trace the symbol effortlessly using the waist to guide the direction of the hand while opening and closing the chest at the proper locations within the symbol.

Rocking. The next set of exercises are performed with one foot forward. For the initial training, if your right foot is forward, use the right hand to trace the symbol. If your left foot is forward, use the left hand. Eventually train with the opposite foot and hand to reach deeper levels of training. Training with one foot forward prepares you for the stepping action used while training two-person symbol exercises. This type of training also conditions the joints of the legs as well as provides a better feeling of rooting when moving forward and backward.

The body, chest, hand, and breathing movements of this exercise remain fundamentally the same as they are when you are standing in the ma bu position. For this particular exercise, coordinate those movements with shifting back and forth between four-six stance (si liu bu, 四六步) and mountain climbing stance (deng shan bu, 登山步) at various sections of the symbol.

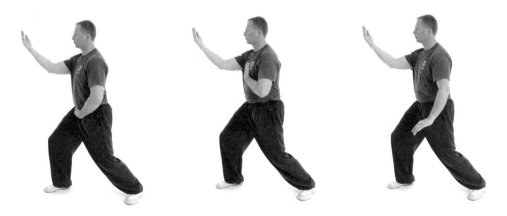

To begin this exercise, use the right hand and stand with the right leg forward. Depending on your intent for training, the left hand may be placed on the lower dan tian, on the center of the chest, or out to the side for balance.

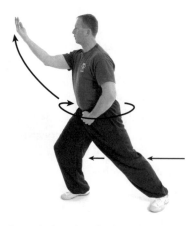
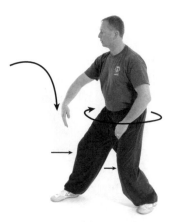

With the right hand in the beginning position, shift back into the four-six stance (si liu bu, 四六步). As the hand traces the outside section of the symbol to the top, shift forward into the mountain climbing stance (deng shan bu, 登山步). As you trace the top outside section of the symbol back down to the bottom, shift your weight back into the four-six stance (si liu bu, 四六步).

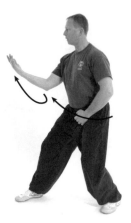
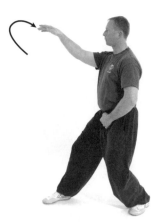

Moving the hand into the center of the symbol from the bottom to the top then into the center of the symbol from top to bottom, you will remain in the four-six stance (si liu bu, 四六步).

When you reach the originating position, repeat the pattern. Practice this exercise until you are able to perform the movements smoothly and continuously throughout the symbol with the proper chest actions. You should also be able to shift your weight back and forth effortlessly while tracing the symbol. Once you have completed this exercise using the right hand, place your left leg forward and practice the exercise with your left hand. Finally, place your right leg forward and repeat the exercise with your left hand.

Stepping. The next exercise to practice is to step forward and backward while practicing the symbol training. This exercise focuses on just one area for the transition to step forward and one to step backward. It should be noted that there are other areas where the transitions are possible. As your skills develop, you will be able to find these other areas on your own. In addition, the symbol you trace while solo is slightly different than with a partner. We will highlight this difference in the two-person training section.

For this exercise, begin in the four-six stance (si liu bu, 四六步) with your right leg forward. Begin to practice the yang vertical symbol training while rocking. While practicing this exercise, it is a good idea to have your nonactive hand placed by your lower dan tian or chest area. This will allow a cleaner transition for the hands. Remember, the symbol is not completely defined as vertical. It has a momentary action of forward and backward traveling of the hand incorporated within it. This will help you in understanding the flow of forward and backward movement.

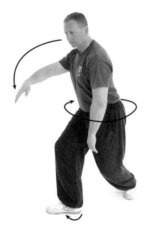

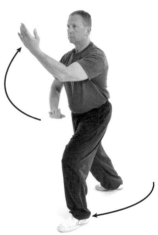

To step forward, wait until your hand is traveling from the bottom outside section of the symbol on up to the top. For this forward movement, transition from your four-six stance (si liu bu, 四六步) into mountain climbing stance (deng shan bu, 登山步). Before reaching the mountain climbing stance (deng shan bu, 登山步), turn your body and forward foot slightly out for the transition. Your hand will reach the top of the symbol and begin to circle down on the opposite outside section of the symbol, palm turning down.

Shifting your weight forward, begin to place the left hand out in front of your body. From this position, you will place your left foot forward and move the left hand forward into your new yang vertical symbol.

The left hand may pass either under the right hand or over the right hand. Practice the transition both ways for application in two-person training. Continue to practice the symbol a few times using the left hand then begin your transition to step forward once again. The procedure is the same for this side. Allow the left hand to circle from the bottom outside section of the symbol to the top while turning your body slightly to the left with the left foot turning out. Shift your weight forward while the left hand continues on its path down around the outside section of the symbol. The right hand will now pass either over or under the left hand and you will now be back practicing the right hand vertical symbol training.

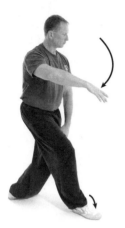

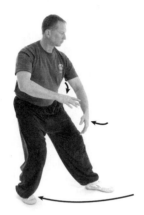

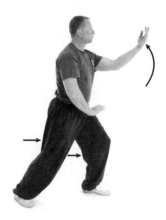

| To step backward, transition as follows. With your right leg forward, practice the vertical yang symbol training with your right hand. From the forward position of the symbol with your right hand on the top of the symbol, begin to shift your weight back while your right hand transitions from the top outside section of the symbol down to the bottom. | Begin to step backward and continue to move your right hand up into the center of the symbol. The left hand will now take over, passing either over the right hand or under. | From this position begin to shift your weight forward for proper execution of the left hand vertical yang symbol training. |

Continue to practice this action and complete a few symbols using the left hand before stepping backward once again. Next, transition back to the right hand. To execute the transition, allow the left hand to circle around the outside section of the symbol to the bottom. While shifting your weight back, place your left foot back and begin to move your right hand out into the symbol.

Continue to practice both the forward and backward movements until you are able to perform the actions in a smooth and continuous flow. You should be able to combine the forward and backward stepping within the same exercise.

Tips to Avoid Common Errors. One of the common errors beginners make while training the vertical yang symbol is turning over the hand too quickly when tracing the outside section of the symbol and transitioning over the top. Allow the hand to pass the vertical plane in front of you before turning the hand over. This will help you keep your shoulder from shrugging and help the elbow stay down, thus allowing the arm to remain fixed with the body movement. Using peng energy while performing the symbol tends to be forgotten as well. Remembering that the symbol is a three-dimensional object and allowing the hand to extend forward and backward throughout the symbol will help the practitioner with opening and closing the chest area and displaying peng energy. When practicing the rocking section of this exercise a common error is to move the hand separately from the body. The hand should reach the top of your symbol at the same time you reach the end of the mountain climbing stance. In addition, don't allow the hand to move around the symbol without twisting your body back and forth.

2. Solo-Horizontal (Dan Lian-Shui Ping, 單練—水平)

Next, the exercise will be performed tracing the symbol horizontally. Once again the thumb will lead the hand throughout the symbol. For this exercise, the closest position will be in front of your dan tian area. The furthest point of the symbol will be arm's length without straightening the elbow. The sides are slightly wider than shoulder width. This is, of course, only for the initial training. As you advance, you can change the height and size of the symbol.

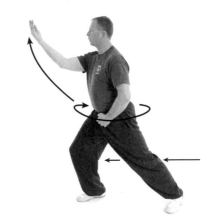

Common error: turning over hand too soon.

Stationary. Stand in the ma bu stance with your right hand in front of your dan tian area, palm facing you.

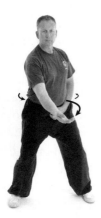

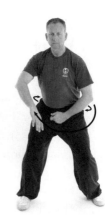

With the chest in the closed position, begin to exhale while you twist your body to the left, moving the hand forward to trace the outside section of the yin-yang symbol. Next, twist your body back to the right while opening your chest and leading your hand around the outside section of the symbol. Your arm will continue to extend out in front of your body while your chest opens and your palm rotates, allowing the thumb to continue to lead the hand around the symbol.

When you reach the farthest point of the circle, begin to inhale and continue to twist your body to the right while you draw the hand back toward you. Close your chest while your hand is drawn back toward your body.

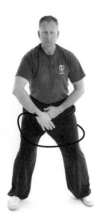

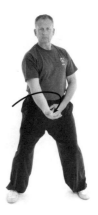

Twist your body back to the left, continue to inhale, and draw the arm back to the original position in front of your body to complete the outside section of the symbol.

Begin to exhale while opening your chest and twisting your body to the left while your hand begins to trace the inside section of the symbol. The palm rotates away from you, and your body turns back to the right as you draw your hand through the center section of the symbol.

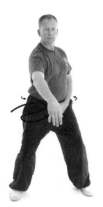 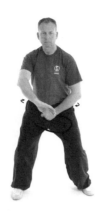 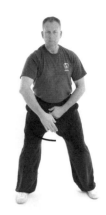

Once the hand has reached the midpoint, continue to twist your body to the right while you open your chest and move your hand out toward the opposite end of the symbol.

Twist back to the left while simultaneously moving the hand around the farthest point of the symbol. The palm rotates back toward you. Now begin to inhale and start closing the chest while you twist your body back to the left and begin to draw the hand from the far outside section of the symbol into the center section.

Your hand passes back through the center of the symbol as you twist back to the right then continues on its path back to the original position while you twist back to the left. End with the palm in front of the dan tian facing forward and the hand facing your body.

Continue to practice this exercise until you are able to execute the movements smoothly.

Once you have completed this exercise using the right hand, practice the horizontal symbol training using your left hand. The circling will move in a counterclockwise direction. The actions are fundamentally the same as for the right hand. Repeat this exercise for the left hand until you are able to trace the symbol effortlessly using the waist to guide the direction of the hand while opening and closing the chest at the proper locations within the symbol.

Rocking. The next stage of practice is to perform the horizontal symbol training with one leg forward. Fundamentally, the body, chest, hand, and breathing movements of this exercise remain the same as they are when you are standing in the ma bu position. For this exercise you will coordinate those movements with shifting back and forth between four-six stance (si liu bu, 四六步) and mountain climbing stance (deng shan bu, 登山步) at various sections of the symbol.

As with all symbol training exercises, you may place your left hand on either the dan tian, chest, next to the opposite elbow, or out to the side. This will depend on your training preference.

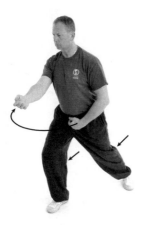

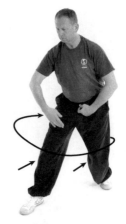

Stand in the four-six stance (si liu bu, 四 六步) with the right leg forward. The right hand will be level with the dan tian, palm facing your body. Begin to trace the outside section of the circle. Moving your hand forward, begin to shift your body forward into the mountain climbing stance (deng shan bu, 登山步). When you reach this position, you will be facing forward with your hand at the most forward position of the symbol.

Next, twist your body back to the right while tracing the opposite outside section of the symbol. At the same time, shift back into the four-six stance (si liu bu, 四 六步). End with your body facing forward and your hand back in front of the dan tian area.

Now you are ready to begin passing through the center of the symbol. Remain in the four-six stance (si liu bu, 四六步) while you first twist your body to the right then left while moving the hand through the center to the most forward position of the symbol. Next, draw the hand back through the center of the symbol while twisting back to the right. End with the hand back at the original position of the symbol while in the four-six stance (si liu bu, 四六步).

Practice until you are able to execute the movements continuously throughout the pattern. Next, practice the exercise using the left hand. Also practice with the left foot forward, using your right hand and then your left.

Stepping. The final sets of exercises for horizontal yang symbol training are the forward and backward stepping exercises. There are more ways to practice these exercises. You are encouraged to create other methods of training. After all, this is an art.

Practicing these stepping exercises is not unlike practicing the vertical stepping exercises. The left hand initially will be placed by your dan tian throughout your practice and then by the armpit area of the hand that is executing the symbol.

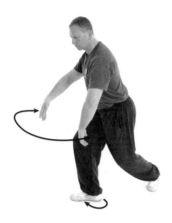
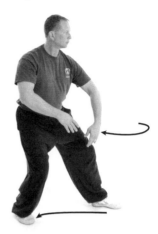

Initially, practice transitioning the forward stepping while your hand is moving forward around the outside section of the symbol.

Backward movement entails your hand moving backward around the outside section of the symbol.

Continue to practice these movements until you are able to step forward and backward smoothly. As with the vertical training, you may find other sections of your symbol where you are able to transition forward or backward. Training with another person will also change the section of the symbol that you transition forward and backward.

Tips to Avoid Common Errors. Common errors that occur when training the yang symbol on the horizontal plane are not unlike the ones that occur on the vertical plane. Simple things to watch for are proper chest movement and making sure the waist guides the hand around the symbol. When rocking forward and backward there tends to be a disconnect in the timing of the hand and body with relation to the area of the symbol. When you are circling around the outside section of the symbol you will want to make sure that your hand reaches the most forward position at the same time your body is at your most forward position. Reaching the most aft position, the hand should be in your most aft position of the symbol. Stepping forward and backward, one must pay attention to keeping the body connected and using the cross leg stance in transition. Initially there tends to be a disconnect between the upper body and lower body when stepping, and the hand performing the symbol training moves without the turning of the waist. With practice this will become less of an error.

2.7.2 Two-Hand Yang Symbol Training

(Shuang Shou Yang Quan Lian Xi, 雙手陽圈練習)

In the next set of exercises you will train using both hands at the same time. This type of training is necessary to train both sides of the mind and body and for engaging an opponent. Just as a concert pianist uses both hands that can react differently, you should be able to utilize both hands when engaging your opponent. Eventually you will train both hands to simultaneously perform a freestyle method of circling where you will be able to exchange between yin and yang effortlessly. This will become more apparent as you engage your opponent and work toward the applications of symbol training. For the following exercises the methods of inhaling and exhaling described may be reversed if you desire. Depending on your choice in size of symbols, your hands may also cross each other as they pass through the various sections of your symbols.

1. Vertical Two-Hand Yang Symbol Training

(Chui Zhi Shuang Shou Yang Quan Lian Xi, 垂直雙手陽圈練習)

Stationary. To practice this exercise, stand in the ma bu position with your arms out in front of your body at waist height.

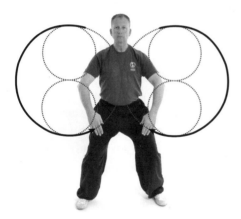

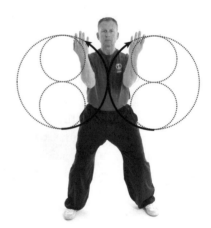

With your body in the wardoff (peng, 掤) posture, begin to exhale, generate the action of movement up through your spine, and circle your arms around the bottom of the yang symbols toward the centerline of your body.

Continue to circle the arms up through the inside section of your symbols.

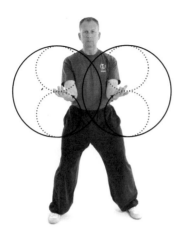

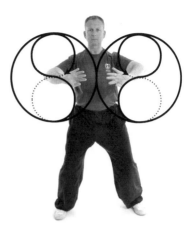

Moving to the top of your symbol, the palms are facing you, your chest is opening, and your arms are moving slightly away from your body. Passing over the top of the symbols, begin to turn the palms over toward the ground while lowering the arms back toward your waist. Continue to lower your hands around the outside section of your symbols while inhaling and closing the chest. Next, circle the hands through your centerline then into the center of each of the symbols.

The spine continues to generate the action while your chest closes and then begins to open again as your hands circle up and through the center of the symbols. You will change from inhaling to exhaling until the hands reach the top of your symbols. Continue the movement with the hands circling up over the top then again passing down through the center of the circle.

The chest will change from opening to closing while the hands circle in to the center of your symbols and you will inhale through this section. Finally, circle the hands back to the starting position while closing the chest and completing the inhalation. Continue to practice this exercise until you are able to continuously generate the action from your body, properly open and close the chest, and complete the symbol without thought. Remember that the thumb generally leads the action throughout the yang symbol.

Rocking. The next stage of exercise is to practice the two-hand yang symbol training. In this exercise you will first practice the two-hand symbol training with the right leg forward then practice it with the left leg forward, all while rocking back and forth. Due to the similarity of this action to the single hand training, we will not describe this in detail here. As with the single hand training, most of the action will be performed while in the aft position of your symbol. You will practice this exercise while rocking back and forth until it becomes smooth and continuous with proper breathing and body movements throughout the symbol.

Stepping. In the final stage of two-hand vertical yang symbol training, begin with the right leg forward while rocking. Then, transition to the left leg forward by stepping forward, all while practicing the symbol training using two hands. In addition, you need to learn to transition backward as well. For your initial practice, we suggest you step forward when your hands move through the inside section of your symbol and step backward when your arms move around the outside section of your symbol. As you become more comfortable with your training, you will be able to find other sections of your symbol for transitioning forward and backward.

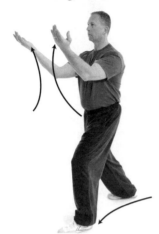 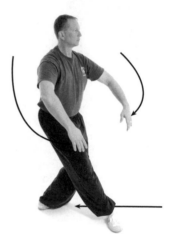

Two-hand vertical yang symbol training pattern with stepping.

Tips to Avoid Common Errors. The most common error is the notion that using two hands at once is difficult. Movement of the two hands at the same time requires a little more effort, but with time you will find it becomes easier. Also, the generation of action from the spine through your body with opening and closing of the chest seems to be a concept students forget to employ. Remember, the hands do not move solely on a vertical plane. They travel forward and backward throughout the symbols. This should help with opening and closing the chest as well as generating the action from the dan tian area up through the spine. Finally, watch the transition when you are stepping forward or backward. The goal is to be able to move forward and backward smoothly while tracing the symbols.

2. Horizontal Two-Hand Yang Symbol Training (Shui Ping Shuang Shou Yang Quan Lian Xi, 水平雙手陽圈練習)

Stationary. This exercise is the two-hand horizontal yang symbol in the stationary position.

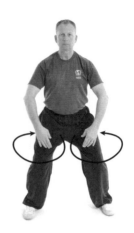

Horizontal two-hand yang symbol training pattern: stationary.

Stand in the ma bu position with your hands placed out in front of your dan tian area. Begin to exhale while you generate the action of movement from your dan tian up the spine and out through the hands. Circle your hands toward your centerline and away from your body. The chest will begin to open as your hands extend forward. Continue to circle the hands around the forward section of the symbols then back toward the body to complete the outside section. As the hands circle back toward you, inhale and close the chest. Next, circle your hands forward and into the center section of the symbols while exhaling and opening your chest. Follow your symbols out of the center section to the far end then circle your hands back into the center section again as you inhale and begin closing the chest. Continue to circle the hands back out of the center of the symbols and return them back to the original starting position while completing the inhaling and closing of the chest. Practice this exercise until you are able to perform the actions with proper body movements generated from the dan tian in a smooth continuous movement.

Rocking. The next exercise is similar to the two-hand vertical yang symbol training. You are simply performing the exercise using the horizontal symbol with two hands while rocking. This will be done with the right leg forward and then the left leg forward. Due to the similarity to the vertical symbol training and single horizontal symbol training, we will not fully describe the exercise here. You should practice this with either leg forward until you are comfortable with the exercise. The movements should be generated by the body and both breathing and chest movements should be continuous throughout the symbol.

Stepping. As with the vertical symbol training, you should also perform this task using the horizontal symbol training with two hands. Due to the similarity of this exercise to the two-hand vertical and single hand horizontal yang symbol training, we will not fully describe the exercise here. For your initial training we recommend you step forward when the hands are circling forward on the inside section of your symbol and step backward while the hands circle around the outside section of your symbol. As you become more comfortable with the exercise, you may find other areas where you are able to step forward and backward. Continue to practice this exercise until you are able to perform it with proper body movements throughout the symbol.

Tips to Avoid Common Errors. The errors commonly made in this exercise are not unlike those in the vertical exercises. The most common is not moving the spine in a continuous wave throughout the symbol. Pay attention to the opening and closing of the chest. As with the vertical symbol training, the horizontal symbol is not entirely made on the horizontal plane. As you become more comfortable with your training, you may increase the height or constantly change the height of the symbol throughout your practice. Finally, be careful of the transition while stepping forward and backward. The forward movement here begins from your most aft position in the symbol. Stepping backward is initiated from the most forward position.

2.7.3 Yin Symbol Training—Solo (Yin Quan Dan Lian, 陰圈單練)

The next set of exercises are the yin side of symbol training. The yang side of training is one half of the necessary symbol training. Without the yin side, your options for effectively neutralizing an incoming force are limited. Training both the yin and yang sides will assist you in a complete understanding of different options of yin and yang neutralizations.

1. Solo-Vertical (Dan Lian-Chui Zhi, 單練－垂直)

Stationary. The following exercise is the yin symbol training while stationary. To begin, stand in the ma bu stance with the right hand placed out in front of your dan tian area, palm facing down. Initially, the left hand will be placed on your dan tian for practice, then later at waist height to your side, and finally up by your right armpit area.

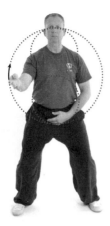

Exhale while twisting your body to the right. Use the waist to generate the action up the spine and out your arm as you raise your hand up along the outside section of the symbol. The pinkie will lead for most of the movement in the yin symbol. Raise your hand away from your body while your chest opens slightly.

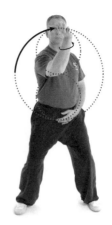

When you reach the top right-hand side of your symbol, rotate your right forearm, turning the palm face up. This will allow the pinkie to continue to lead the yin symbol. Next, begin to inhale, drop the right elbow, close the chest, and twist your body to the left as you move your hand over the top of the symbol down around the left hand side.

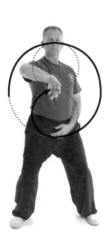

Once your hand reaches the original starting position, begin to move your hand through the center section of the symbol. Twist your body slightly to the right then back to the left while you exhale and begin to open the chest.

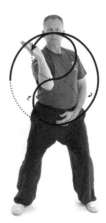

Allow the hand to grow away from your body while passing through the center and out to the top of the symbol. Now follow through the center of the symbol again by twisting slightly to the right and back to the left while you inhale and close the chest.

Twist your body back to the right and allow your right hand to return to the original starting position. Continue to practice until you are able to execute the yin symbol with the proper body movements throughout the exercise.

Rocking. The next step is to practice the yin symbol training using the rocking method. Practice with your right leg forward and then with your left leg forward. To begin, stand in four-six stance (si liu bu, 四六步) with your right leg forward. Your right hand is placed out in front of the dan tian and your left hand is on the dan tian. Later you will practice with the left hand out to the side and then up by your right armpit area.

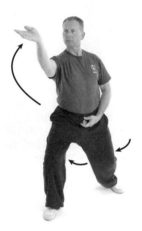

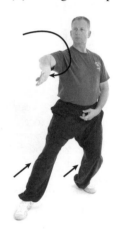

Exhale and shift your weight forward into mountain climbing stance (deng shan bu, 登山步) while you move the action up your spine, open your chest, and raise your right hand up along the right side of the symbol.

Rotate the right palm up, begin to inhale, and continue to move the hand over the top of the symbol down the left-hand side. Shift your weight aft into four-six stance (si liu bu, 四六步) while this occurs. From this position, remain in the four-six stance (si liu bu, 四六步) while you follow the symbol through both center sections.

Once you have completed the symbol, shift back into the mountain climbing stance (deng shan bu, 登山步) while your hand continues on to the next symbol. Continue to practice this until you are comfortable with the coordination of rocking and proper body movements while executing the symbol. Include training with the left hand out to the side and also by your right armpit area. Next, place your left leg forward and practice the yin symbol for the opposite hand.

Stepping. The next exercise involves stepping while practicing the yin vertical symbol. To properly execute this exchange of hands while stepping, you may find it easier to place the non-active hand back by the armpit area of the hand performing the symbol. Once again there are multiple areas to exchange hands in the symbol. We only demonstrate one area.

Once you have stepped forward, continue to practice the yin vertical symbol with the opposite hand while rocking. After tracing the symbol a few times, step forward again.

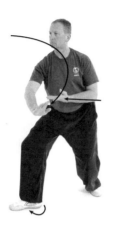

To begin, stand in four-six stance (si liu bu, 四六步), right leg forward. Practice the yin vertical symbol training with your right hand while rocking. To step forward, allow your right hand to circle down along the right outside section of your symbol. Then slide the left hand either over or under the right arm while stepping forward.

Again, the symbol is not completely linear. You can expand and withdraw within the symbol. Eventually your training will combine the symbols, creating nothing but a sphere.

While rocking, you will want to be sure to coordinate your forward and aft movement with the tracing of the symbol. While stepping, your initial concern will be the coordination of the symbol and the forward or backward movement of stepping itself.

You will end with the opposite leg forward and the opposite hand now tracing the yin symbol vertically. Continue to practice stepping forward and backward until are you are comfortable with performing the exchange. The movements should be a continuous flow throughout the transition. Remember that the transition is only explained in one spot here. You are encouraged to explore other areas of the symbol to execute your stepping.

Tips to Avoid Common Errors. Common errors for the yin single hand training are similar to those of yang training. Remember to open and close the chest while waving the spine throughout the symbol.

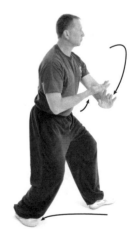

Next, practice stepping backward. In order to practice this step, continue with your current symbol training until you reach the most forward section of your symbol. Your hand tracing the symbol will be traveling over the top and down the outside section of the symbol. Begin to shift your weight back while the hand travels further down the outside section of your symbol. The hand tracing your symbol travels back as the opposite hand travels forward, taking over the symbol tracing.

2. Solo—Horizontal (Dan Lian—Shui Ping, 單練一水平)

The next set of exercises involves practicing the single hand yin symbol in a horizontal manner. For these exercises, the placement of the hand not actively tracing the symbol initially will be placed by the lower dan tian, then to the side for balance, and finally by the armpit of the hand that is performing the symbol. Initially, the size of the symbol will be as follows: the farthest end of the symbol will be such that the elbow of the arm is not locked while the hand is extended in front of your body. The sides will be approximately shoulder width apart. Once you are comfortable with this, you may change the size of the symbol as well as the height or angle of the symbol. Additionally, breathing will be described along with chest movements for each section. You may elect to inhale and exhale at sections of the symbol different than what we have described in each section.

Stationary. To begin training the horizontal single hand yin symbol, start in the stationary position.

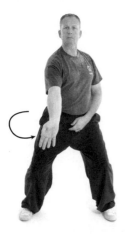
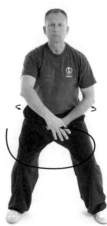

Stand in the ma bu stance with your right hand out in front of your dan tian. In the beginning, practice with your left palm on your dan tian, then with your left hand out to the side, and finally with it up by the right armpit. Initiate your movement up through your spine, out your arm, and into your hand so that the hand begins its path around the outside section of the symbol to its most forward section. You will be exhaling while your chest initially opens.

As you reach the farthest point of the symbol, twist your waist and lead your right hand around the other side back toward your body. Inhale and close the chest while your hand approaches your body. Twisting back to the forward facing position, begin to exhale, open your chest, and lead your hand back through the center of the symbol out to the far end.

Continuing with the pattern, draw your hand back through the symbol while closing the chest and inhaling. This should bring you back to your original starting position. From this position, continue to practice the symbol until you are able to perform the actions with the proper body movements throughout the symbol. Once you are comfortable with this, change to the left hand and continue with the symbol for the left side.

Rocking. The next sets of exercises are the rocking exercises that are performed while practicing the single hand horizontal yin symbol.

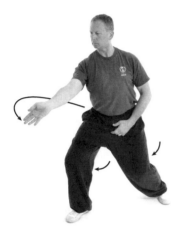

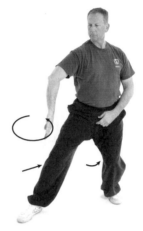

Stand in the siu liu bu position with the right leg forward. Inhale deeply then exhale. As you exhale begin twisting your waist to the right, shift your weight forward in to mountain climbing stance (deng shan bu, 登山步), and move the hand along the outside section of the symbol to its most forward position.

Twisting your body back to the left, draw the hand back around the outside section of the symbol toward you while you shift your weight back into four-six stance (si liu bu, 四六步), closing your chest and inhaling. Remain in the aft position and exhale, open the chest, and move the hand through the center of the symbol out to the far end.

Continue to follow the movement back through the center of the symbol, returning to the original starting point. Practice this exercise until you are able to trace the symbol with the proper body movements. Once you are comfortable with this action, switch the forward leg to the other one and practice the horizontal yin symbol with your left hand.

Stepping. The next set of exercises will be done while stepping. To begin, place your right leg forward and begin your yin symbol training with the right hand. Your left hand should be placed either by your lower dan tian or by the right armpit area. Practice a few symbols before stepping forward. Remember, there are multiple areas in the symbol where you may transition forward and backward. We are using only one area to demonstrate the transition.

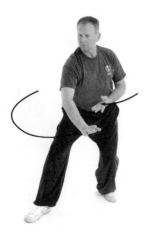 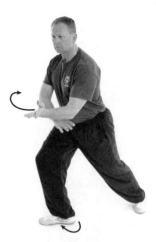

When you step forward, your right hand will be moving over the top outer section of the sym-bol. As your right hand passes around the top section of the symbol and returns back toward you, step forward and extend the left hand for transitioning to the left hand yin symbol.

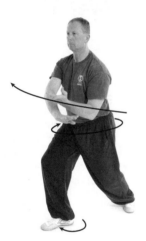 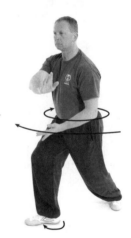

Slide the left hand either over the right arm for diagonal flying (xie fei shi, 斜飛勢) or under the right arm for Grasp Sparrow's Tail (lan que wei, 攔雀尾).

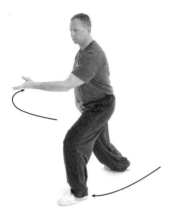 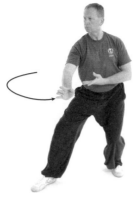 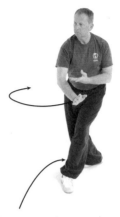

Continue to practice a few symbols using the left hand then step forward once again to transition to the right hand.

Next, practice stepping backward. In this example, the location of the transition will be from the top section of the symbol down along the outside section.

To execute this action, start by practicing a few yin symbols with your right hand and right leg forward. As your hand moves toward the center of the symbol, over the top, and then down along the outside section, begin to step back while moving the left hand forward.

Your left hand will now take over, and you will practice a few yin symbols for the left side. Next, step back again to change to the right side again. Changing hands will occur while you circle up over the top to the outside section. Continue to practice stepping forward and backward until you are able to do so comfortably with the proper movements.

Tips to Avoid Common Errors. The common errors here are similar to the previous errors in both yang vertical and horizontal training. Chest, spine, and transitions are the common fault areas. As you continue to train these exercises, the correct movements become more familiar to your body.

2.7.4 Two-Hand Yin Symbol Training

(Shuan Shou Yin Quan Lian Xi, 雙手陰圈練習)

The next set of exercises are performed with both hands simultaneously. This is accomplished on both the vertical and horizontal plane. The purpose of this type of training becomes more obvious when engaging an opponent. You learn to be cognizant of being able to attach and stick with your opponent with both hands throughout the exchange. Being able to do so with both hands allows you to increase your chance of defeating your opponent.

1. Vertical Two-Hand Yin Symbol Training

(Chui Zhi Shuang Shou Yin Quan Lian Xi, 垂直雙手陰圈練習)

Stationary. The first exercise of the two-hand yin symbol training is tracing the symbol on the vertical plane while stationary.

Reaching the original starting point of your symbols, inhale and draw the hands up through the center of your symbol until they reach the tops then begin to exhale while you circle the hands back through the center of the symbol until you reach your original staring point. Continue to practice this symbol training until you are able to perform the movements with proper breathing throughout the symbols.

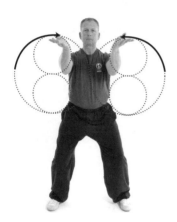

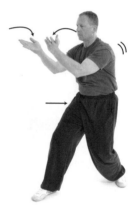

Stand in the ma bu position with both your hands out in front of your lower dan tian. With the palms slightly facing your body, inhale and move your hands up along the outside section of the symbols. As in all the movements, this action begins from the lower dan tian area and rolls up the spine and out into the arms. Circle your arms up on the outside section of your symbol then begin to move your arms down the inside section of the symbols while exhaling.

Begin to inhale while you rock forward and move your hands up along the outside section of the symbols. The action should be initiated from your waist area and carried along the spine out into your arms. As you reach the top of the symbols, shift back into your four-six stance (si liu bu, 四六步) while exhaling and circling the hands back around the insides of the symbols.

Rocking. The next exercise is vertical two-hand yin symbol training while rocking. Stand in the four-six stance (si liu bu, 四六步) with your right leg forward. Place both hands in front of your lower dan tian area.

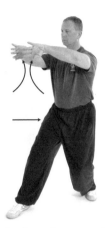
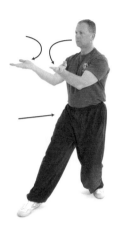

Remain in the four-six stance (si liu bu, 四六步). Inhale and move the hands through the center of the symbols up to the tops. Exhale and draw the hands back through the centers, again ending in the original starting position of the symbols.

From this position you may repeat the symbol training. Practice this exercise until you are able to perform the actions continuously with proper body movements. The location of inhaling and exhaling may be changed if you wish. Once you can do this exercise comfortably, place your left leg forward to practice.

Stepping. The next exercise is to perform the two-hand vertical yin training while stepping forward and backward. Yin solo training while stepping has characteristics similar to yang solo training while stepping. In both cases the symbol is completely traced for both sides while you practice solo. Practicing with a partner will change the way you perform the symbol. This action will be discussed in more detail in a later section.

To practice this exercise, stand in the four-six stance (si liu bu, 四六步) with your right leg forward. With both hands placed out in front of your lower dan tian, begin to perform the vertical yin circling while rocking just as you have done in the previous section.

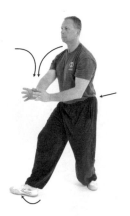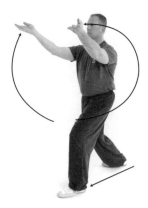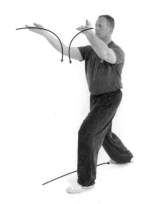

To transition forward, turn your forward foot out slightly, shift the weight forward, and allow the hands to follow the outside sections of the symbol, circling over the top and down toward the centerline of your body.

Slide the left leg forward and continue to trace the symbol while rocking for a few repetitions before stepping forward again.

Once you are comfortable with moving forward, practice moving backward. To step back, simply reverse your direction while the hands once again move over the top of the symbols down into the inside sections.

Continue to practice stepping backward then combine the forward and aft movement until you are comfortable with the transition.

Tips to Avoid Common Errors. Common errors are similar to those previously discussed. Spine, chest, and transitions are among the priorities here.

2. Horizontal Two-Hand Yin Symbol Training

(Shui Pin Shuang Shou Yin Quan Lian Xi, 水平雙手陰圈練習)

Stationary. The next exercise is the horizontal yin symbol training with two hands in the stationary position.

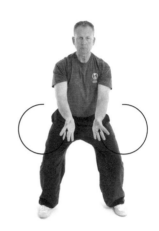

Inhale and draw the hands toward your body, tracing the inside sections of the symbols. Once the hands reach the origination point, you will lead them back through the center sections of the symbol just as you did in the vertical symbols. Be sure to breathe as well as open and close the chest accordingly. Continue to practice this exercise until you are able to execute the movements correctly in a continuous flow throughout the symbols.

Rocking. Next practice the two-hand horizontal yin symbol training while rocking.

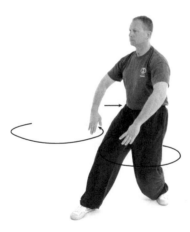

Stand in the ma bu position with both of your hands out in front of your lower dan tian area. Inhale and draw the qi up through your spine. When the qi reaches the dazhui (Gv-14) (大椎) cavity, exhale and begin to move both hands out around the outer sections of the symbols. The chest will close while you continue to move the hands around the far end of your symbols.

Step into the four-six stance (si liu bu, 四六步) with the right leg forward. With the hands placed out in front of the lower dan tian, begin to inhale and lead the qi from your lower dan tian out and up your spine. When you reach your dazhui cavity, exhale, close the chest, and lead the hands around the outer section of your symbols while rocking forward into the mountain climbing stance (deng shan bu, 登山步). Reaching the farthest section of your symbols, turn the palms over, begin to inhale, open the chest, and lead the hands back toward your body while rocking aft.

Once your hands have arrived at the starting point, lead them back through the center sections of your symbols. While the hands move forward through the center of the symbols, rock forward. Drawing the hands back toward your body, rock aft. Continue to practice this exercise until you are able to execute the actions correctly throughout the symbol training. Once you have completed this task, stop and switch your stance so that your left leg is forward and practice it on the opposite side.

Stepping. The next step is to practice the two-hand horizontal yin training while stepping. Only one transition area is explained. There are other areas to transition forward that you should explore on your own.

Practice stepping forward until you are able to make the transition smoothly. Next practice stepping backward. Once again, we only describe one area to practice this transition. We implore you to practice and explore other areas for transitioning back. To step back you will begin in the most forward section of the symbol. As you inhale and move your hands around the inside section of the symbols, step back. Continue to rock back and forth a few times before transitioning back again.

Practice this exercise until you are comfortable with stepping back. The movements should be coordinated with both the hands and legs. As you become more comfortable you will want to practice taking more than one step while stepping.

Tips to Avoid Common Errors. The common errors to watch for while practicing the two-hand horizontal yin training are similar to those found in previous sections. Chest, spine, and transitions should be some of the priorities to be concerned with.

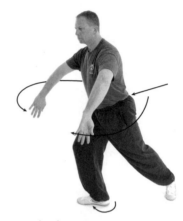

Step into the four-six stance (si liu bu, 四六步) with the right leg forward. Place both hands out in front of the lower dan tian. Inhale and draw your qi up through your spine. When you reach the dazhui cavity, exhale and shift your weight forward into the mountain climbing stance (deng shan bu, 登山步) while moving your hands around the outer section of the yin symbols. Inhale and rock back while drawing your hands back around the inside sections of the symbols. Continue to trace the symbols while rocking until you have reached the original starting point. To step forward, turn your right foot out slightly while in the aft position. Step forward while exhaling and circling your arms around the outside section of the yin symbols.

2.7.5 Mixed Training—Yin-Yang Two-Hand Training

(Yin Yang Quan Shuang Shou Hun He Lian Xi, 陰陽圈雙手混合練習)

Once you are comfortable with both yin and yang two-hand training, practice the same set of exercises with one hand performing the yang symbol while the other simultaneously performs the yin symbol.

Use the instructions already provided and practice training while stationary, rocking, and stepping.

Once you are comfortable using opposite symbols on either hand, practice performing an exchange for the hands within the symbols. For example, the left hand is performing the yang symbol while the right hand is performing the yin symbol. While you are doing the symbols, change so that the left hand changes to the yin symbol and the right hand changes to the yang symbol. There are endless combinations to practice. This type of training will allow you to exchange more quickly while you are engaging your opponent in two-hand pushing hands.

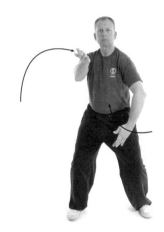

To begin this training, start with both hands out in front of the lower dan tian. As you gain skill you will be able to start the symbol in different areas of the symbols.

2.7.6 Two-Person Single-Hand Yin-Yang Symbol Training—Yang

(Yin-Yang Taiji Quan Shuang Lian—Yang, 陰陽太極圈雙練—陽)

The next stage of training yin-yang symbol training requires a partner. Training with a partner is important in developing connecting, listening, adhering, attaching, and following jing skills. Also, having a partner helps you learn the proper amount of pressure to apply to another person in single and double pushing hands training. Finally, you and your partner will experience various degrees of being double-weighted while stepping forward and backward. Double weighting occurs when there is no distinction between that which is insubstantial and substantial force. There is an increased amount of pressure between you and your partner, which in some cases may cause a bump in the fluid motion through the symbol. This usually occurs when there is a breakdown in the listening and following skills between you and your partner. These exercises will be described using vertical symbol movements followed by horizontal movements, and then combining them.

1. Vertical, Yang (Chui Zhi—Yang, 垂直一陽)

Stationary. The first stage of practicing the single hand yang vertical two-person symbol training is stationary. Face your partner in the ma bu stance and trace the symbol. Although your body movements are similar to the solo practice, there are some differences in tracing the actual symbol when working with a partner.

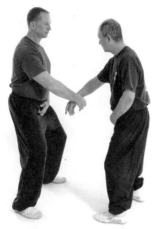

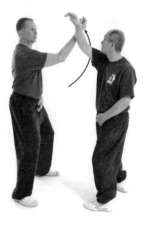

Stand in ma bu facing your partner with your hands facing toward your dan tian. Touch together the inside sections of your wrists.

The inside and outside wrist area will be the main region of contact throughout the exercise. Begin to trace your symbol as you normally have done while practicing solo.

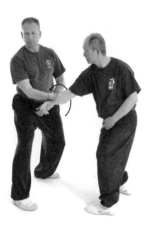

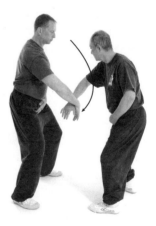

Your partner will follow your action with their hand as you complete the outer section of the symbol. Next, you begin tracing the inside section of the symbol just as you did in the solo practice.

When you reach the center section of the symbol, also known as the wuji point, your partner takes over the action of tracing the symbol and you follow his motion. The hand continues to trace through the center section of the symbol then over the top of the symbol and continues on the outside section of the symbol to the left until you reach the original starting point.

From this position, your hand moves into the center section of the symbol where you will again take over the action of tracing the symbol. With your partner now following your action, move the hand out of the center of the symbol to the top. From this position, repeat the actions as previously described. This exercise should be practiced until you both are able to move continuously throughout the symbol. Once you have accomplished this repeat the action for the opposite hand.

Rocking. The next exercise involves rocking while practicing the single hand yin-yang symbol.

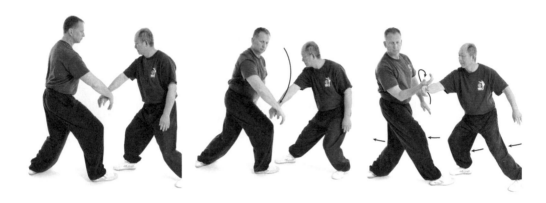

Face your partner with your right feet forward. Interlock your hands. To begin the symbol training, you will both be in a neutral position with your weight distributed equally on both legs.

Start tracing the symbol as you did while stationary. Rock forward into the mountain climbing stance (deng shan bu, 登山步) while tracing the outside section of the symbol up to the top. Your partner rocks back into the four-six stance (si liu bu, 四六步).

Passing over the top of the symbol to the right bottom outside section, begin to rock back.

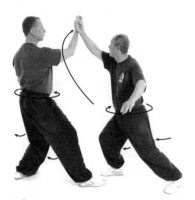

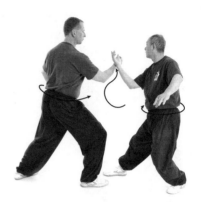

Next, move your right hand up through the center of the symbol, shifting fully into the four-six stance (si liu bu, 四六步).

Remain in the four-six stance until you have passed your hand through the center of the symbol, over the top, around the left outside section, and back down to the bottom of the symbol.

Reaching this point, you repeat the previous action with your partner. Continue to practice this exercise until you can both do it smoothly, then repeat the action for the opposite hand with the left leg forward.

Stepping. The next stage of vertical training involves stepping while performing the yang side of single hand yin-yang symbol training. There are two stages of training this exercise. The first stage is to training the sense of distance. In this stage you will step forward and backward while maintaining an equal distance between you and your partner while you both train the symbol.

Your partner needs to sense the forward action and slides their right foot back in order to step backward accordingly. Continue to practice the symbol while stepping forward as space allows then have your partner step forward. As you both become comfortable with this procedure, you can start to move forward and backward more freely. With this training each of you are attempting to catch the other off guard and cause the opposite person to lose balance or be sealed when you move forward. Continue to practice until you are able to move forward and backward smoothly. Once you have done this, train the opposite side.

The second stage of this exercise involves the exchange of the dominant hand of symbol training.

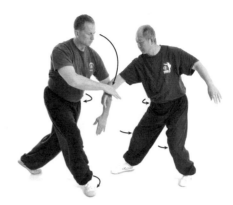

Stand facing your partner with right legs forward. Interlock hands and begin to trace the symbol just as you did in the rocking position. To transition to the opposite side, start from your most aft position with your hand on the bottom of the symbol. Turn the forward foot outward and circle the right hand through the center and over the top of the symbol then begin a path down on the outside section of the symbol.

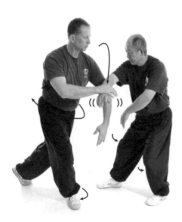

Shift your weight onto your forward foot as your left hand begins to intercept your partner's right arm.

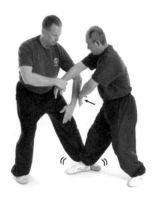

Slide your left foot forward placing it behind your partners right foot to trap it. Your partner will intercept your left arm and will be moving the right foot back to avoid this trap.

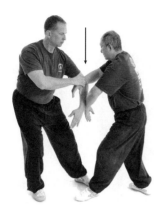

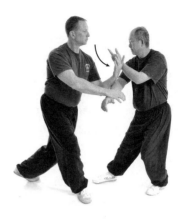

This interception is followed by one of two methods. One, the left hand continues under your partner's right arm thereby performing the technique of Grasp Sparrow's Tail (lan que wei, 攔雀尾).

Two, the left hand can continue to move above your partner's right arm performing Diagonal Flying (xie fei shi, 斜飛勢).

Both interceptions are applied while simultaneously stepping the left foot forward. In a more combative exercise the goal is to place the left foot directly behind your opponent's forward foot. This, however, is a training exercise, which means your partner knows your next move and simultaneously steps back while intercepting your left hand with their left hand. You both retract your right arms as the change to the left hands continues. If you don't retract your right arms, they will be trapped. Continue to practice a few rocking movements before stepping forward once more.

As you become more comfortable with stepping forward, allow your partner to step forward a few times. This training develops your sensitivity to adhering, listening, and following jing. The idea is to maintain the same pressure throughout the stepping process and not cause a bumping sensation. If you find you are having difficulty with exchanging hands, go back to stationary training and practice exchanging hands without stepping.

Tips to Avoid Common Errors. The common errors for the two-person single hand vertical yang symbol training are similar to those of solo practice. Watch for your body, waist, and chest to properly move while performing the symbol. It is important to remember the nature of the exercise and do not apply too much force on your partner. Although you may be moving forward in your symbol, you still need to listen to your opponent's energy. This two-person training exercise is the base that will assist you with the neutralization exercises in later sections.

2. Horizontal (Shui Ping, 水平)

Stationary. The first stage of practicing the single hand horizontal two-person symbol training is performed while stationary.

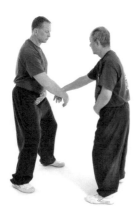

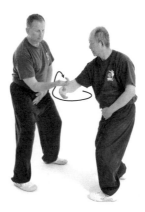

Face your partner in the ma bu stance while tracing the symbol. Place your right hand out in front of you with the left hand on your lower dan tian. Your partner's right hand touches yours and their left hand is on their lower dan tian. The inside sections of your wrists should be touching.

The inside and outside wrist area will be the main region of contact throughout the exercise. Begin to trace the symbol as you have done while practicing solo. Your partner follows your action with their hand as you complete the outer section of the symbol. Next, you begin tracing the inside section of the symbol similar to your movement in solo practice.

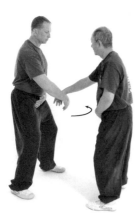

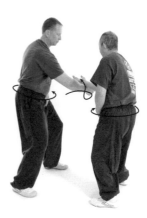

Your hand continues to trace through the center section of the symbol then around the far outside section of the symbol to the left until you reach the original starting point.

Now your hand moves back into the center section of the symbol then out toward the outside far section, repeating the actions as previously described.

This exercise should be practiced until you both are able to move continuously throughout the symbol.

Rocking. The next exercise is to practice the single hand horizontal yin-yang symbol while rocking.

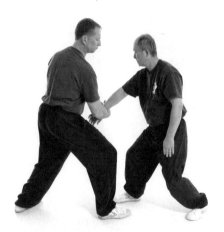

Face your partner with your right legs forward. Interlock hands. To begin the symbol training you both are in a neutral position with weight disturbed equally over both legs.

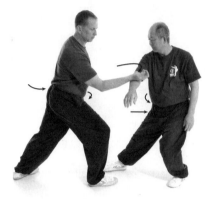

Start tracing the outside section of the symbol. You rock forward into the mountain climbing stance (deng shan bu, 登山步) while your partner rocks back into the four-six stance (si liu bu, 四六步).

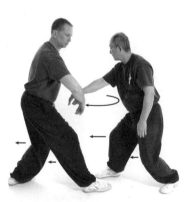

Begin to rock back while passing around the forward section of the symbol to the original position. Passing through the center of the symbol, shift fully into the four-six stance (si liu bu, 四六步).

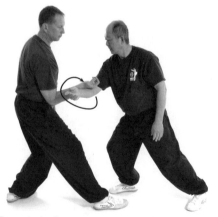

Remain in four-six stance until you have passed through the center, forward section, left outside section, and back to the original section of the symbol.

Reaching this point, you rock forward into the mountain climbing stance (deng shan bu, 登山步) while moving the hand back through the center. Continue to practice this exercise until both you and your partner are able to execute the movements smoothly.

Stepping. The next stage of single hand horizontal yin-yang symbol training is to practice this exercise while stepping. This training is similar to vertical stepping training. It also has two stages of training. In the first stage you and your partner step forward and backward while tracing the symbol on a horizontal path. Again, the idea is to catch your partner off balance and seal or trap their movements to allow an attack.

To begin this training, face your partner with your right legs forward. Begin the horizontal symbol training while rocking. To step forward, turn the forward foot out while in the aft position then step forward while circling the hand forward on the outside left section of the symbol. Continue to step forward as space allows then allow your partner to practice stepping forward. Once you are both comfortable, you should move freely forward and backward. Each time either one of you steps forward you are attempting to catch the other one off guard and seal their arm. The person who is stepping back is focusing on maintaining an equal distance throughout the move-

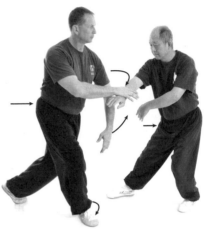

Two-person single hand horizontal yang symbol training pattern with stepping.

ment. Once you both are comfortable with practice this exercise, exchange to the opposite hand and repeat the exercise.

The second stage of this exercise involves exchanging the dominant hand when you step forward and backward. To begin this exercise, stand facing your partner with the right legs forward. Interlock your right hands and begin to practice the horizontal single hand yin-yang symbol training while rocking. To step forward and exchange your dominant hand, begin from the aft position with your right hand tracing the left outside area of the symbol. Turn the forward foot out and begin to shift your weight forward onto the right foot. The hand continues around the forward section of the symbol while the left hand begins to move toward your partner's right elbow. Your left foot should slide up to and behind your partner's right foot in an attempt to trap it. They in turn will slide their right foot back and begin to intercept you left hand in order to continue tracing the symbol. From this position, you will now practice the single hand yang symbol training using your left hand. Continue to practice this side a few times before attempting to step on to the opposite side. After you have practiced stepping, your partner should then practice stepping while you move aft.

Once you are both comfortable doing the exercises, practice the stepping techniques in a more freestyle manner where either individual may elect to move forward. In this stage you must both listen more carefully to the other person in order to avoid any bumping in force.

Tips to Avoid Common Errors. The common errors that occur in the horizontal single hand two-person yang training are similar to those of the vertical training. Make sure the chest and waist movements guide the arm throughout the symbol. Additionally, watch for using too much force or overextending yourselves. When your partner steps forward you must also be aware of bumping or double weighting and learn not to become sealed while stepped upon.

2.7.7 Two-Person Single Hand Yin-Yang Symbol Training—Yin

In this section, we will discuss the two-person single hand yin symbol training. This will allow you to increase your options for neutralization when engaging your opponent. Without this training you are limiting yourself to half of the necessary components of listening, following, adhering, and controlling jings. The following training will be described while stationary, rocking, and stepping both vertically and horizontally.

Stationary. The first exercise is the two-person single hand vertical yin training in the stationary position.

Reaching the bottom of the symbol, your partner will begin his attack by rotating his palm up and circling through the center of the symbol. As you pass through the center of the circle, begin to coil your hand over your partner's right wrist and circle from the top of the symbol along the outside section to the bottom. Notice that you are now tracing one half of the symbol you were originally tracing while solo; this is similar to what you have done in the yang section of training. Practice this action until both you and your partner are able to completely trace the symbol without causing a bumping sensation between you. Once you are both comfortable performing this exercise, change to the left hand and repeat the exercise.

To begin this exercise face your partner in the ma bu position with your right hands touching at the wrist. Your partner begins to attack by circling up and over the top of the symbol. You initiate your movement up your spine, out your arm, and into your hand. Neutralize your partner's incoming force by coiling over their wrist with your right hand and trace your symbol around the left outside section to the bottom of the symbol.

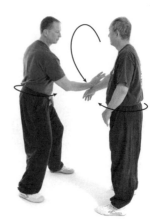

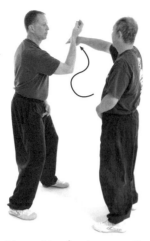

From this position begin your attack by turning your wrist palm up and following through the center section of the symbol up to the top.

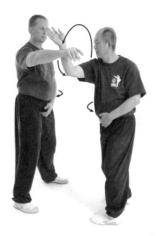

Your partner follows this motion and begins his neutralization by coiling over your wrist and redirecting your action over the top of the symbol down around the outside section of his symbol.

Rocking. The next stage of the two-person single hand yin symbol on a vertical plane training is to practice the exercise while rocking.

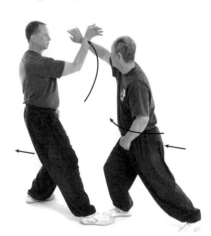

Face your partner with your right legs forward. Place your right wrist on your partner's right wrist. Starting from your most forward position follow your partner's forward action and lead his hand over the top section of the symbol down along the left hand side to the bottom section of the symbol. This is coordinated with shifting the weight aft.

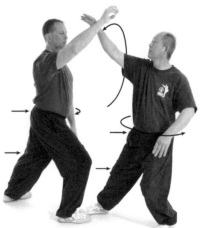

When you reach the bottom section, turn the right hand over and begin to pass through the center of the symbol while shifting forward again. Your partner will coil over your right hand and begin to lead your forward action over the top of the symbol down along the opposite side of the symbol until it reaches the bottom.

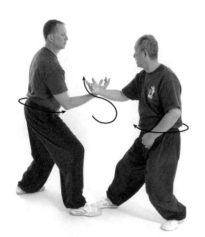

Next, your partner turns their hand palm facing up and begins their attack forward.

Now lead your hand up through the center of the symbol, coil over your partner's right hand, and lead their forward attack over the top of the symbol down along the side to the bottom. Repeat this exercise back and forth until you and your partner are able to rock back and forth smoothly and continuously while tracing the yin symbol. Once you have completed the exercise for the right hand, change to the left hand with the left leg forward.

Stepping. The next exercise is the single hand yin vertical symbol training with exchanging hands while stepping. This process is similar to the yang side of stepping exercises. Use either of two techniques in order to exchange hands while stepping: Grasp Sparrows Tail (lan que wei, 攔雀尾) and "diagonal flying" (xie fei shi, 斜飛勢). Practice using only one of the techniques, then move on to the other technique before mixing the two techniques.

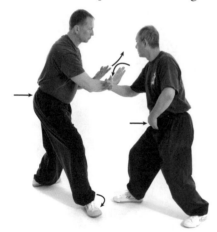

Stand facing your partner with your right legs forward. Interlock your right hands and start the single hand vertical yin training while rocking. To step forward and exchange hands, turn your right foot out while your weight is aft and your right hand is circling down along the left hand side of your symbol. As your right hand travels toward the bottom of your symbol, begin to shift your weight forward while sliding your left hand forward over your right hand to execute diagonal flying (xie fei shi, 斜飛勢).

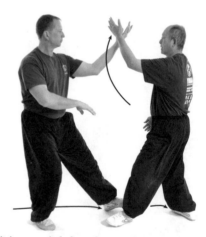

Slide your left foot forward in an attempt to trap your partner's right foot. They will slide their right leg back, avoiding the locking of the leg while extending their left hand to intercept your left arm.

From this position rock back and forth a few times before attempting to step forward again. Practice stepping forward until you reach the end of your practice area then allow your partner to practice stepping forward. Once you are both comfortable stepping forward and backward, practice the exercise using a freestyle method of stepping forward and backward. Continue to practice this exercise until both of you are able to step forward and backward smoothly while exchanging hands.

Practice rocking a few times with the left leg forward then step forward again. Reaching the end of your practice area, have your partner practice stepping forward using the same hand. Once you have both stepped forward and backward, you may swap to the left hand and practice the same stepping techniques for the opposite side.

Tips to Avoid Common Errors. The common errors in this section are similar to those of the yang side of training. Body movements including chest, spine, and breathing while moving through the symbol should be natural. One concern on the yin side is to be sure to slide along your partner's arm while stepping forward. It is necessary to follow your partner's arm in order to prevent your partner from being able to strike you. You should also be aware of the trapping of the foot when you advance as well as when you withdraw.

2.7.8. Vertical/Horizontal/Two Hand Training—Two Person
(Chui Zhi/Shui Ping Shuang Shou Dui Lian, 垂直水平雙手對練)

In the following exercises, you will practice both the yin and yang sides of symbol training using both hands while training with your partner. These exercises are done while in the stationary position as well as in the rocking and stepping positions. They can be practiced both in the vertical and horizontal planes as well. We recommend you practice the movements performing the yang side first then the yin side. After you and your partner are comfortable, you may select, exchanging from yang to yin or yin to yang. At this stage of training you should be comfortable with performing the symbols both in the yang and yin side using single and double hands.

2.7.9 Freestyle/Mixed Training
(Zi You Hun He Lian Xi, 自由混合練習)

The last training exercise for the partnered symbol training is freestyle/mixed training. In these exercises you are going to exchange one or both hands from yang to yin or yin to yang throughout your symbols. This training allows you to enhance your following, listening, adhering, and attaching skills. You and your partner will practice this while in the stationary position as well as in the rocking and stepping positions. At this point you should be comfortable with performing the yin-yang symbols in the vertical and horizontal planes while in the stationary, rocking, and stepping positions.

References

1. "其根在腳，發於腿，主宰於腰，形於手指。由腳而腿而腰，總須完整一氣。向前退後，乃能得機得勢。Dr. Yang, Jwing-Ming, *Tai Chi Secrets of the Ancient Masters* (Wolfeboro, NH: YMAA Publication Center, 1999), 3–4.

2. Dr. Yang, Jwing-Ming, *Taijiquan Theory of Dr. Yang, Jwing-Ming* (Wolfeboro, NH: YMAA Publication Center, 2003), 180.

3. 立如平準，活似車輪。Dr. Yang, Jwing-Ming, *Tai Chi Secrets of the Ancient Masters* (Wolfeboro, NH: YMAA Publication Center, 1999), 20.

4. "身形腰頂皆可以 ，粘、黏、連、隨意氣均。Dr. Yang, Jwing-Ming, *Tai Chi Secrets of the Yang Style* (太極拳楊氏先哲祕要), (Wolfeboro, NH: YMAA Publication Center, 2001), 50.

5. Dr. Yang, Jwing-Ming, *Tai Chi Secrets of the Yang Style* (太極拳楊氏先哲祕要), 47.

6. "拿住丹田練內功，哼哈二氣妙無窮。"乾隆舊抄本歌訣。 Dr. Yang, Jwing-Ming, *Tai Chi Secrets of the Yang Style* (太極拳楊氏先哲祕要), 77.

7. "喉頭為第二主宰。"太極拳之三要論。 Dr. Yang, Jwing-Ming, *Tai Chi Secrets of the Yang Style,* (太極拳楊氏先哲祕要), 43.

8. "有上即有下，有前即有後，有左即有右。Dr. Yang, Jwing-Ming, *Tai Chi Secrets of the Ancient Masters,* 7.

9. Dr. Yang, Jwing-Ming, *Taijiquan Theory of Dr. Yang, Jwing-Ming,* 110.

10. "力由脊發。""牽動往來氣貼背，而練入脊骨。Dr. Yang, Jwing-Ming, *Tai Chi Secrets of the Wǔ and Li Style* (太極拳武、李氏先哲祕要) (Wolfeboro, NH: YMAA Publication Center, 2001), 7, 10.

11. Yang, Jwing-Ming, *Taijiquan Theory of Dr. Yang, Jwing-Ming,* 115–117.

12. "手足相隨腰腿整，引進落空妙如神。Dr. Yang, Jwing-Ming, *Tai Chi Secrets of the Wǔ and Li Style* (太極拳武、李氏先哲祕要), 36.

13. Dr. Yang, Jwing-Ming, *Taijiquan Theory of Dr. Yang, Jwing-Ming,* 186–188.

Chapter 3: Taiji Jing Practice

3.1 Introduction

Jing (勁) or martial power training is an important part of the Chinese martial arts, but there is very little written on the subject in English. Theoretically, jing can be defined as "using the concentrated mind to lead the qi to energize the muscles and thus manifest the power to its maximum level." From this, you can see that jing is related to the training of the mind and qi. That means qigong (氣功).

Traditionally, many masters have viewed the higher levels of jing as a secret that should be passed down only to a few trusted students. Almost all Asian martial styles train jing. The differences lie in the depth to which jing is understood, in the different kinds of jing trained, and in the range and characteristics of the emphasized jings. For example, tiger claw (hu zhua, 虎爪) style emphasizes hard and strong jing, imitating the tiger's muscular strength; muscles predominate in most of the techniques. White crane (bai he, 白鶴), dragon (long xing, 龍形), and snake (she xing, 蛇形) are softer styles, and the muscles are used relatively less. In taijiquan (太極拳) and liu he ba fa (六合八法), the softest styles, soft jing is especially emphasized and muscle usage is cut down to a minimum.

The application of jing brings us to a major difference between the Oriental martial arts and those of the West. Oriental martial arts traditionally emphasize the training of jing, whereas this concept and training approach is relatively unknown in other parts of the world. In China, martial styles and martial artists are judged by their jing. How deeply is jing understood and how well is it applied? How strong and effective is it, and how is it coordinated with martial technique? When martial artists perform their art without jing it is called "flower fist and brocade leg" (hua quan xiu tui, 花拳繡腿). This is to scoff at the martial artist without jing who is weak like a flower and soft like brocade. Like dancing, their art is beautiful but not useful. It is also said, "Train quan and not gong, when you get old, all emptiness."[1] This means that if a martial artist emphasizes only the beauty and smoothness of his forms and doesn't train his gong, then when he gets old, he will have nothing. The "gong" here means "qigong" (氣功) and refers to the cultivation of qi and its coordination with jing to develop the latter to its maximum and to make the techniques effective and alive. Therefore, if martial artists learn their art without training their "qigong" and "jing gong" (勁功), once they get old the techniques they have learned will be useless because they will have lost their muscular strength.

Often jing has been considered a secret transmission in Chinese martial arts society. This is so not only because it was not revealed to most students, but also because it cannot be passed down with words alone. Jing must be experienced. It is said that the master "passes down jing." Once you feel jing done by your master, you know what is meant and can work on it by yourself. Without an experienced master it is more difficult, but not impossible, to learn about jing. There are general principles and training methods that an experienced martial artist can use to grasp the keys of this practice. If you are interested in this rather substantial subject, please refer to the book: *Tai Chi Chuan Martial Power,* by YMAA Publication Center.

In this section we will describe various jing patterns you may use as a foundation for listening, understanding, attaching, sticking, connecting and following. Before you begin these movements, you need to be sure to properly warm up your body. If you train jing, especially soft jing, you should be aware of possible injuries if you are not cautions. We will discuss how to prevent injury in the next section.

Breathing and the yi also need to be coordinated to properly manifest jing. For each of the following jing patterns, you may choose to move slowly first then pick up the speed of the action as your body becomes more comfortable with the movements.

3.2 Injury Prevention

When you train jing, you must be very careful, especially during soft jing training. This is because when you are emitting a strong jing outward, your ligaments and tendons at the joints will be pulled strongly and instantly. It is common to be able to grasp the key of emitting jing (fa jing, 發勁) in a short time. However, it takes a long period of time and correct methods to condition your joints so they are able to bear the sharp and sudden pulling.

Here are a few important keys for your jing training that can prevent a lot of unnecessary injuries.

1. Condition joints. Condition your joints before you train your jing patterns, especially soft jing. Condition means to strengthen the structure of the joints including ligaments, tendons, bones, and any other structure related to endurance and strength. The places that need to be conditioned are the spine, shoulders, elbows, and wrists. The most common places for injury are the spine, shoulders, and elbows. Therefore, the conditioning exercises should be designed especially for these joints. White crane qigong is specially designed for this purpose. After you have mastered all of these qigong movements, then you should hold some weight in your hands, starting with one pound and then increase to five pounds when joints are stronger. If you are interested in this conditioning, please refer to the book and DVD: *White Crane Qigong*, by YMAA Publication Center.

2. Find an experienced and qualified teacher. It is said in Chinese martial arts society that "jing can only be passed by a master individually." This is because jing cannot be seen easily. The manifestation of jing should be felt. A qualified master will be able to direct you to these feelings correctly. Once you have established these feelings, you can then practice by yourself. This is especially true when soft jing is trained.

3. Train body structure and root. Without correct body structure and a firm root, injuries can occur. Furthermore, in order to manifest your jing efficiently and powerfully, you must have a few firm foundations. In Chinese martial arts society, it is recognized that the body acquires six bows (liu gong, 六弓) that allow you to store the power and then manifest it. These six bows include spine, chest, both legs, and both arms, though some styles consider that the spine and chest (i.e., torso) should be treated as one bow. You must learn how to coordinate these six bows and manifest your power from your legs through your torso and finally in your hands. In *Taijiquan Classic*, it is said, "Once in motion, every part of the body is light and agile and must be threaded together."[2] Also it is said, "The root is at the feet, jing is generated from the legs, controlled by the waist, and expressed by the fingers. From the feet to the legs to the waist must be integrated, and one unified qi."[3] From these statements, you can see that soft jing's manifestation should be executed as a soft whip. In addition, you will also need a firm root. Without a firm root, you will not be able to manifest your jing powerfully.

4. Train hard jing before soft jing. When hard jings are manifested, the body is stiffer. That means the joints are locked. When the joints are locked, the pulling power to the joints is at a minimum. Thus, less damage or injury is likely to occur. Usually, it is the correct way of training a beginner. Only after the joints are conditioned should soft-hard jing be trained. In soft-hard jing training, the body is soft and relaxed first. When the qi has reached to the arms, then the body is tensed for manifestation. That means when the power reaches the end for manifestation, the joints are also tensed and thus protected. Soft jings are the hardest to train since you don't tense the joints when power is manifested. However, you must know the timing for rebounding backward. When you have caught the right timing of rebounding the whip backward, you prevent the ligaments and tendons from pulling. It is difficult to master the trick of soft jing. A qualified teacher will be able to direct you to the correct way of practice.

5. Train short jing before long jing. This is especially true for soft jing training. When you manifest jing for a short range, you must bounce your power backward before the arms are completely extended, thereby protecting the joints. Only when your joints are stronger and endurable, and the timing of your rebounding is correct, should you then gradually increase the long jings' training.

6. Train no more than thirty minutes per day. This is especially true for a beginner. If you train correctly, just thirty minutes of jing training puts your ligaments and tendons in a tolerant situation. If you continue, you may injure yourself. An experienced martial artist should pay attention to the condition of the joints and adjust the time of training.

7. Rest. After training, you need rest. Your ligaments, muscles, and tendons will be sore. Rest and allow them to recover. Do not allow your ego to take over the training. Overdoing the training to sooth your ego often leads to injury. If you like you may do some gentle movements. Gentle joint movements enhance the blood and qi circulation. This will expedite the recovering process.

8. If you're already injured, rest and let it heal. If you find that pain from injury persists, see a good doctor. It often takes a few months for the body to heal the injury. Prevention from injury is the key of long-lasting training.

3.3 Basic Jing Patterns for Taijiquan Pushing Training

The following jing patterns are basic jing training techniques for taijiquan training.

1. Double Push Jing (Shuang Tui Jing, 雙推勁)

For the first training exercise, stand in the ma bu position with your hands placed approximately at your waist, shoulder width apart.

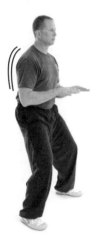
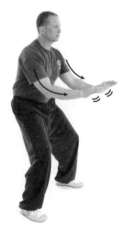

Begin to inhale while initiating the action of movement from the feet up into the waist then up the spine, out through the shoulders, and into the hands.

It should feel as though a wave has started in the waist and traveled all the way up your spine, through the arms, and out the hands. Exhale when the action has reached the shoulders and you begin to continue the action through the hands. As the power is manifested through the hands, sink your body slightly into the feet.

Your hands should remain at waist height until you are comfortable with this waving action, then you may begin to raise the hands higher. Continue to practice this action until you are able emit the jing comfortably through the hands while they are at shoulder height.

The next stage is to practice the pattern while standing with one foot placed forward. An important note: you must not lock the rear leg when executing this jing pattern. This soft jing action is generated from the legs so they must also be loose. Place the right leg forward and stand in a four-six stance (si liu bu, 四六步). Begin to inhale while drawing the action up through the rear leg into the waist. The action then moves from the waist, up through the spine, across the shoulders along the arms, and out the hands. Exhale as it passes the shoulders and travels out the hands. Continue to practice this movement with the hands at waist height until it becomes comfortable then continue to raise the hands up for each jing. The final stage of jing manifestation is at shoulder height.

Tips to Avoid Common Errors. Common errors often involve shrugging the shoulders when you begin to raise the arms to shoulder height. Shrugging your shoulders causes energy stagnation throughout the neck and often results in pain occurring in the neck. There are also common tendencies to float up when performing the exercise. Sink your body when manifesting the jing. Finally, remember the action is a whipping action. The hands should snap back toward your body. If you find you are having problems with this, there are a few ways to correct it. First, return the arms to the lowest position and practice the jing pattern at this level. Second, you may break down the action further by practicing this movement slower at all the levels. This will allow the body to learn the movements more accurately.

2. Single Push Linking Jing (Dan Tui Lian Huan Jing, 單推連環勁)

In this exercise execute the jing with one hand.

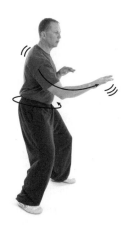 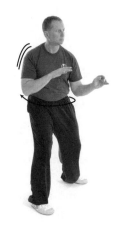 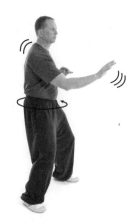

Stand in ma bu and place the hands at waist level. Inhale and initiate the action up through the legs into the waist. From this position begin to twist the waist in order to load or chamber the first action of jing.	Exhale, twist the waist in the other direction, and allow the first hand to move forward for the first jing. This allows the second jing to load or chamber.	Finally, continue to exhale while you twist the waist back and allow the second hand to move forward and execute the jing.

Keep in mind that your waving action is still occurring through the spine while you twist back and forth.

Tips to Avoid Common Errors. Commons errors to watch for are the tendency to shrug your shoulder as you raise the arms higher. There is also an incorrect tendency to float when executing this jing. Make sure you sink into the feet when executing this type of jing. You should also be sure to wave the spine along with opening and closing the chest. This is how the power is able to manifest itself further.

3. Splitting Jing (Lie Jing, 捋勁)

The next jing to be practiced is the splitting jing. This action is shown in the taijiquan movements known as Grasp Sparrow's Tail to the left (zuo lan que wei, 左攔雀尾) and diagonal flying (xie fei shi, 斜飛勢). The action of splitting jing is that of two opposing forces.

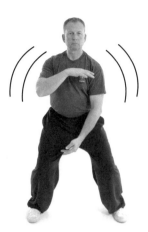

To practice this jing, stand in your ma bu stance with one hand placed palm up in front of your lower dan tian area. Place the opposite hand, palm down, near the chest.

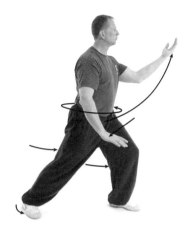

Inhale while closing the chest and creating your wardoff (peng, 掤) posture. This assists you in compressing and storing the jing. Turn out the foot of the lower hand and prepare to emit your splitting jing. Begin to exhale while simultaneously twisting the waist, shifting the weight toward the forward foot, diagonally moving the hands away from each other and opening the chest. The upper hand ends with the palm facing you at approximately the same height as your face while the lower hand ends palm facing down and approximately waist height.

From this position, turn the lower hand palm up while turning the opposite hand palm down. Once again assume the wardoff position and begin to inhale for storing the jing. Shift the weight aft slightly and turn your body back toward the ma bu position. This will allow you to turn the recent forward foot back to the forward-facing position and reset your body for applying the action to the opposite side. Once this has been done, you may turn the opposite foot out and execute the same pattern of jing movements to the other side.

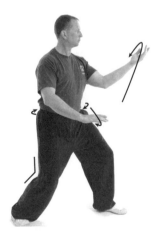

Immediately following the execution of jing, allow your body to relax and return to a neutral position.

Tips to Avoid Common Errors. First, do not lean your body forward when closing the chest and storing the jing. Second, be sure to turn the waist when emitting the jing action. Make sure both arms move in opposite directions. One hand is used for attacking an opponent while the other is for balance. Also be careful of floating. There is a tendency for practitioners to rise when executing the jing because the body tends to follow the arm moving upward. To correct this action, remember to sink your body when twisting into the forward leg. Finally, be aware of the movement being one continuous flow from bottom to top. This means that when you emit the jing the body expands together as one unit. Once the jing has been emitted, the body returns to the neutral position. Remember this is a soft jing similar to a whip. The most common error when emitting jing through a mountain climbing stance (登山步) is the tendency to forget the legs and remain in this stance while allowing the upper body to return to the neutral position. The lower body must return to a neutral position as well. To avoid this stagnation, practice the movements slowly then increase the action until you are able to execute this jing fluidly throughout the entire body and return to a neutral position.

4. Wardoff Jing (Peng Jing, 掤勁)

The next jing pattern is known as wardoff jing (peng jing, 掤勁). Of the Thirteen Postures of taijiquan practice, wardoff (peng, 掤) is the first and foremost posture. Peng is necessary for yielding and neutralizing, and it is also part of the essence of storing jing. Wardoff (peng, 掤) is present throughout the taijiquan sequence. We will present just a few of the wardoff jing (peng jing, 掤勁) patterns you may practice. As you become more comfortable and more aware, you may elect to add or change the angles of the wardoff jing (peng jing, 掤勁).

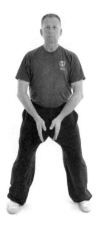

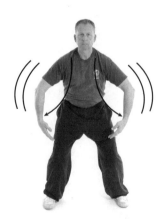

In order to practice the first wardoff jing (peng jing, 掤勁) pattern, begin by standing in the ma bu stance. Inhale while opening your chest slightly. With the arms down by your sides, draw them in slightly.

Next, exhale and begin to draw the energy up through the legs, into the spine, then out through the arms. The arms move out away from your body while closing the chest.

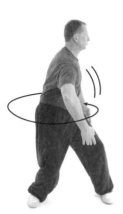

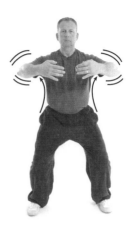

In each execution of this jing, your body must sink into your root. Practice this action for a few repetitions then change the angle by twisting the waist side to side. To perform this movement, simultaneously twist your body to one side while you exhale, expand arms out to the sides, and close the chest.

After a few repetitions, raise the arms so the hands are approximately chest level and repeat the actions of wardoff jing (peng jing, 掤勁).

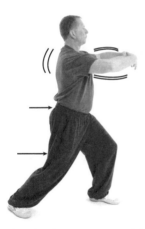

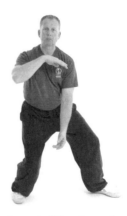

Next, stand in the four-six stance (si liu bu, 四六步) and practice the wardoff jing (peng jing, 掤勁) forward and to your sides. Begin with the arms arcing downward first then raise the arms to approximately chest level. Practice until you are comfortable then switch the stance so the other leg is forward. Repeat the pattern.

For the final wardoff jing (peng jing, 掤勁) pattern, place one hand approximately chest level, palm facing down. Place the opposite arm down by the waist. Begin to inhale and close the chest to store the jing.

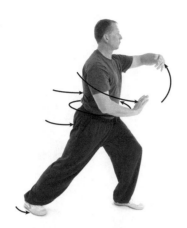

To execute the jing, begin to exhale while drawing the energy up through the foot. Shift the weight forward and twist the waist. The hand that was at chest height moves downward as the lower arm moves up to approximately chest height. The chest will open up at this point. The hand that moves downward does so at an angle. It is not a straight vertical movement. The hand moves similar to that of the push (an, 按) or settle the wrist movement as it goes forward.

Tips to Avoid Common Errors. When executing wardoff jing (peng jing, 掤勁), do not shrug your shoulders up toward your neck. Some students also lose their root when executing the jing. One of the most important mistakes is forgetting to draw in the chest and arch the back, also known as the oral secret "han xiong ba bei" (含胸拔背). This movement is used to properly store jing in the chest and spine. One must also learn how to manifest jing efficiently through the coordination of the legs, waist, spine, chest, and arms. Be mindful of your lower body in executing these jings when shifting into a mountain climbing stance (登山步). The entire body must return to a neutral position. Finally, as with all jing patterns, you need to have the sense of enemy when practicing the jing patterns. This helps in the manifestation of the jing pattern and give meaning to the action.

5. Pressing Jing (Ji Jing, 擠勁)

The next jing pattern is pressing jing (ji jing, 擠勁). This jing pattern is best for short-range fighting. It is generally used as an offensive maneuver with the intent to either destroy your opponent's central equilibrium or attack cavities.

We describe both the pressing and squeezing aspects of this jing in the following exercises.

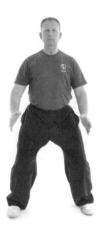

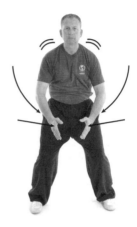

To begin the press jing (ji jing, 擠勁), stand in the ma bu stance with your hands placed in front of your waistline. Inhale while opening the chest and condensing the jing.

Next, exhale sink your body while closing the chest, and compress the arms together slightly. The movement feels as though you are squeezing a beach ball in front of your body. Repeat the exercise until you are comfortable with the pattern.

Next, practice the jing pattern while you twist your body from side to side.

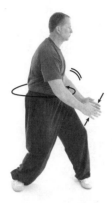 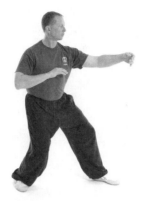 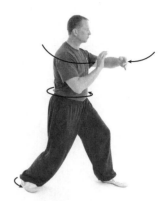

Stand in the ma bu stance, chest open and arms to the sides. To execute the jing movement, twist your body to one side while exhaling, closing the chest and compressing the arms inward. Practice until you feel comfortable.

Change to the four-six stance (si liu bu, 四六步) stance. From this position practice the same action a few times. Include the twisting of the waist. Next, change the position of your hands. The left hand or right hand may be placed so the arm is parallel to the ground with the palm facing toward you while the opposite hand is placed in front of your chest area, palm facing toward the other hand.

Inhale, open the chest, and condense the qi for the jing. Exhale, close the chest, and compress your body while moving the two hands toward each other in a squeezing motion. Practice this action until it is smooth and rooted through the feet.

Next, change to the pressing movements.

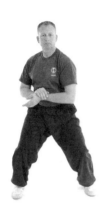 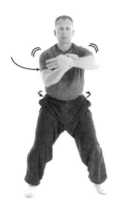 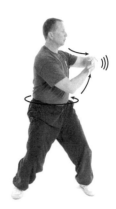

Begin in the ma bu stance. Place your right hand on the wrist of the left, twist your body to your right, and bring the hands down toward the waist area of your body. This is done simultaneously as you inhale, close the chest, and condense the jing.

Exhale while twisting the waist back to your left and pressing the hands diagonally up and away from your body. The chest will open as the hands move in this direction. Continue these movements for a few repetitions then change hands to practice this action for the opposite side.

As you become comfortable with this pattern, train the jing pattern while twisting your body to the left and right. Begin with inhaling, twisting your waist to your side, and drawing your hands down to your waist. To execute the jing, exhale, twist your waist completely to one side, and diagonally raise the arms up chest level.

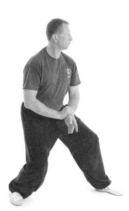 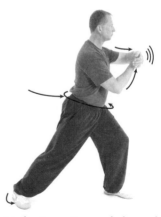

Once you have trained this jing in the ma bu position, step into the four-six stance (si liu bu, 四六步) for the next exercise. The hands will begin down in front of the waist and the torso will be slightly turned away from the front leg. Inhale, close the chest, and condense the jing in your body.

To execute the jing action, exhale, push off the rear foot, twist the waist, open the chest, and raise the arms up and away from your body. The hand of the rear leg will be pressing the wrist of the opposite hand. The arm of the forward leg will end with the forearm parallel to the ground.

Once you have executed this action, immediately relax your body back into a neutral state. Continue to practice this pattern until you are able to execute the jing correctly.

Tips to Avoid Common Errors. One of the most common errors lies with rooting. Be sure to sink your body into your root when executing the jing. Along with the sinking, avoid sticking out the butt and do not lean forward when extending the arms. The waist needs to turn for directional power manifestation, especially while executing the jing in the four-six stance (si liu bu, 四六步) to mountain climbing stance (deng shan bu, 登山步) transition. The chest will need to open and close to store and manifest the jing. You also need to have the sense of enemy to assist in placing the manifestation of jing beyond the area of your movement.

6. Twisting Jing (Niu Zhuan jing, 扭轉勁)

The next jing pattern is the twisting jing. Twisting jing is an important jing in taijiquan training, especially for pushing hands. When facing an opponent, it is necessary to twist your body while applying a technique to uproot the person.

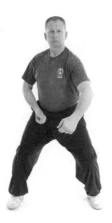

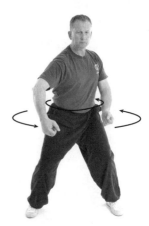

Begin in the ma bu stance. Place your hands at waist height with one hand away from your body and the other close to your body. Inhale and close the chest.

To manifest the jing, exhale, open the chest, and twist the waist while circling the hands to the opposite positions. The movement is similar to turning a large steering wheel on a bus. The hands stay at waist height throughout the maneuver. The sound used while executing the jing is the heng (哼) sound. The reason for this is that you are manifesting jing but you are also conserving jing as well. You do not want to manifest all the power out. 167

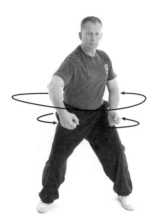
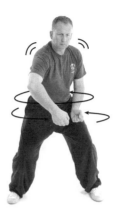

Once you have practiced this jing for a few repetitions, practice the same motion with your chest, closing when you twist. Then practice this jing moving the hands on a diagonal path. Practice the jing patterns with either opening the chest or closing the chest at the end of each movement. Different applications will warrant the chest opening or closing at the end of the action.

Next, practice this jing pattern with one leg forward.

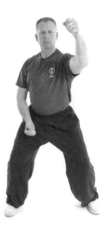

The diagonal movement is executed the same as before; however, the hand that begins closest to the waist will now end out in front of your body at chest height.

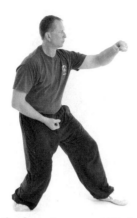

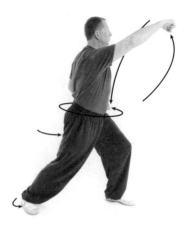

Stand in the four-six stance (si liu bu, 四六步) position and place the hands at waist height in preparation for the exercise. Inhale, close the chest, and condense the jing.

Exhale, twist the waist while you open the chest, and move the hands to the opposite positions.

This exercise should be practiced with the right hand twisting up diagonally while shifting forward as well as with the left hand twisting up diagonally shifting backward. Then practice the same pattern with the opposite leg forward in the four-six stance (si liu bu, 四六步).

Tips to Avoid Common Errors. A common error is not staying rooted to ground. You need to sink your body while twisting. In addition, the twisting action needs to be carried through both hands simultaneously. There is an incorrect tendency for the action of the hand moving toward your body not to follow the twisting action as much as the hand that moves away from your body. You need to focus on the hands acting together as one unit. The waist drives this action.

3.4 Coiling and Spiraling Training

In the next section we will describe the exercises for coiling and spiraling training. The main purpose for training these movements is to enhance the fundamental skills of adhering, connecting, following, and listening. You will also learn to develop your growing jing skills as you spiral from one joint to the next. Growing jing is an offensive jing where you continually grow into your opponent for attacking with a quick, short jing. The mind is focused on approaching and attacking the opponent and thus leads the qi deep into the opponent. As the defender, you will be using all the aforementioned skills as well. You will learn that the spiraling technique is not just a forward maneuver but may be applied backward as well for neutralizing and countering attacks.

Stationary. In the first coiling and spiraling training, stand facing your partner with right legs forward.

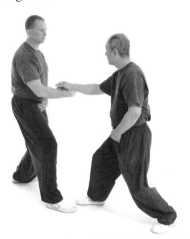

Both of you will place the left hand on the lower dan tian and the right hand out in front of your body touching each other's wrist.

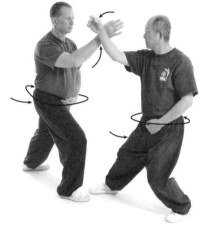

Inhale and begin to twist your body while coiling clockwise over the partner's wrist. From this position, exhale, open the chest, and rock forward while turning the waist and spiraling your hand clockwise toward your partner's elbow.

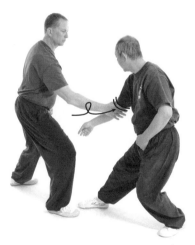

As you are growing into your partner, he will inhale, turn his waist, close the chest, and spiral counterclockwise along your hand while rocking backward. You will end the forward position with your hand on the inside of your partner's elbow for plucking.

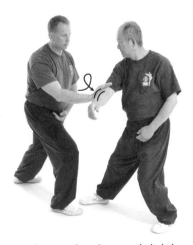

Alternatively, your hand can coil slightly on top of your partner's elbow for sealing.

The spiraling action may be completed to the elbow in one or two movements depending on how quickly you grow into your partner's center. Keep in mind that the more movements you make in a real situation, the easier it will be for your opponent to react and evade your attack. To continue the exercise, your partner must now twist your body with the closed chest, continue to coil the arm with your body, and begin their forward movement while spiraling toward your elbow. Continue this exercise until you are both able to do the movements continuously back and forth. As you both become more comfortable with the movements, focus on spiraling up to the shoulder. Next, alternate between the elbow

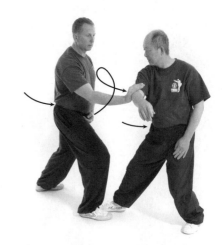

Or, on the outside of your partner's elbow for sealing.

and shoulder in a freestyle manner. Additionally, you should change the size of the movement from circling to spiraling and coiling as well as change the placement of the left hand from the lower dan tian to the side of your body for balance. Once you have done this, exchange sides so that now you are spiraling in a counterclockwise manner and your partner is spiraling clockwise. Finally, practice with the opposite leg forward and repeat the same movements as before.

1. Same Side (Tong Bian, 同邊)

Next, practice the same exercise by placing your left leg forward. Your partner will place their right foot forward.

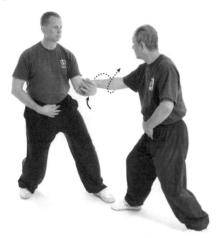

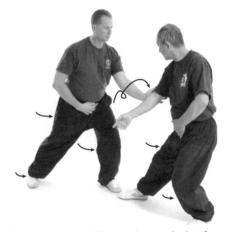

Connect your left wrist with your partner's right wrist.

Your partner will keep their right leg forward throughout this exercise. The movements are the same as before: spiraling each time up to the partner's elbow while rocking forward and spiraling back as your opponent moves toward you.

Practice this exercise until the movements are smooth with correct breathing and chest movements. Be sure to practice it in both directions then place opposite legs forward and practice the movements once again for both directions.

Tips to Avoid Common Errors. Be aware to make proper use of the chest while moving forward and backward. The body needs to twist throughout the movements, especially to avoid the possibility of the arm being sealed against your body. Do not try to change the direction of the movement once it has started.

2. Moving (Dong Bu, 動步)

This exercise is broken down into various subsections. The first stage is to practice in a stationary stance.

Stand in the ma bu stance facing your partner. Place the right hand up against your opponent's right wrist and begin the spiraling movements as previously described in the coiling and spiraling techniques. The left hand may be placed on the dan tian, out to the side, or next to the right elbow.

Next, change the acting arm to the opposite one. The direction of the movement will not change. If you are moving clockwise, continue in that direction. After completing the technique, change hands once again. Once you are comfortable with this action, your partner may begin exchanging hands. Finally, you both can change back and forth between hands while coiling and spiraling.

The next stage is exchanging hands while stepping. Once again you need to focus on stepping to a proper angle to advance into your opponent's central and empty door.

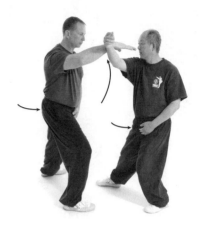

Begin in the mountain climbing stance (deng shan bu, 登山步) with your right leg forward. Begin the same coiling and spiraling exercise as before. This time begin to spiral toward your partner while stepping either to the left or right to enter into their empty door.

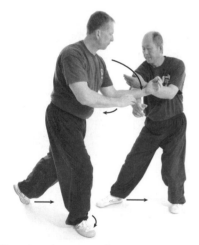
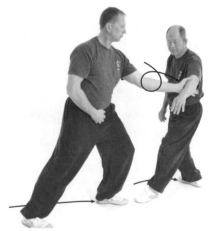

Entering the empty door, your partner will begin to neutralize the advance by stepping, turning your body, and coiling or spiraling back into your empty door by stepping forward either to the left or right.

3. Changing Directions (Huan Bian, 換邊)

The next exercise involves the actual changing of the direction of spiraling and coiling from clockwise to counterclockwise and back while stepping. This is also performed while changing from one hand to the other. The idea is to change the direction of the spiraling action in a smooth and continuous pattern. Do not bring the movement to an actual stop. In order to do this correctly, you need to rotate your body and change the direction of the action through the use of a yin-yang exchange. To execute this maneuver, use the image of the yin-yang symbol that was used in the yin-yang symbol training section. To change directions, move into the center of the symbol, through the center or wuji point, then exit out and continue your action in the opposite direction. Depending on your initial direction, you will notice an S shape or reverse S shape when you pass through the center of the symbol. Keep in mind that the shape of the symbol will be elongated when performing the technique in this exercise.

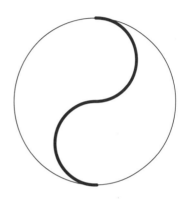

Yin/Yang symbol exchange. moving through the center of symbol to change the direction of movement without stopping the action.

To apply this to the spiraling and coiling training, begin the same exercise of spiraling and coiling while stepping.

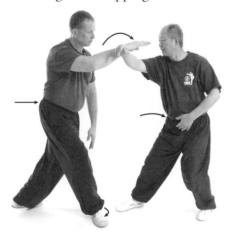

To change the direction, begin to spiral toward your partner's elbow. Step to the side of your opponent, rotate your body, and begin to move your partner's arm through the center of the yin-yang symbol.

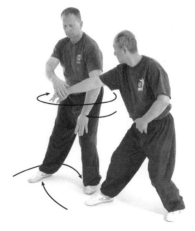

Take your opposite arm and intercept your partner's arm near the elbow.

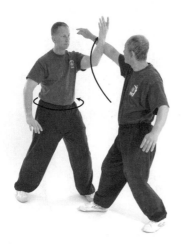 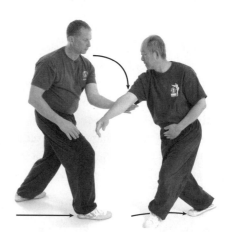

Coiling and spiraling training: changing direction with stepping.

Allow this intercepting arm to continue the movement through the center of your symbol. This action will now flow out of the center of the circle and continue in the opposite direction. Your partner will of course be stepping back while turning their body in order to avoid being trapped. They then continue to spiral and coil while stepping toward your empty door. In order to simplify the exercise you may elect to have one person practice the exchange first then the opposite person. Finally, each person may execute the exchange back and forth in a freestyle manner. Continue to practice this exercise until you are both able to execute the exchange smoothly using the correct body movements. This includes focusing on the proper stepping techniques toward each person's empty door.

3.5 Listening and Following Training

The next exercises are listening and following jing patterns. These exercises will further assist you in training the attaching, listening, following, and adhering jings. You and your partner will practice these exercises using single hand, cross side, and same side actions both in stationary and stepping positions. You will then follow this with double hand training in both the stationary and stepping positions.

1. Single Hand (Dan Shou, 單手)

The first exercise is the single hand listening and following exercise. You and your partner will use cross side training followed by same side training. Both actions will be performed stationary followed by stepping.

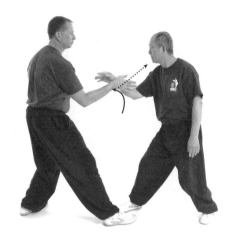

To begin this exercise you and your partner stand facing each other with right legs forward. Attach your right wrist to your partner's right wrist. Next, attempt to coil around your partner's wrist using either a yang or yin coiling, and redirect your partner's limb in an attempt to open an area for you to attack your partner.

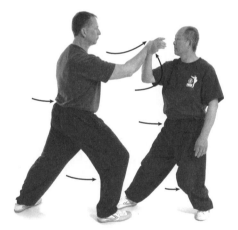
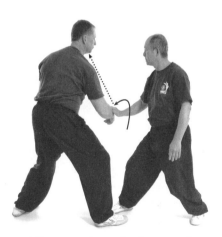

As you begin your forward movement, your partner must follow your incoming force, redirect it, and use a yang or yin coiling technique to get inside or on top of your arm.

Once they have neutralized your incoming force, they will immediately redirect their action to attack you. You will then repeat your action of sticking with their limb following the initial attacking force, redirecting it, then performing the same coiling movement, yin or yang, to begin the process of opening up an area for attack. Continue to practice this exercise back and forth until you are both able to do this smoothly and continuously.

This should also be practiced while the eyes are closed. Once you complete this, swap legs and practice this exercise for the left hand.

The next stage is to practice the exercise while stepping. Begin with the right leg forward and attach the right hands as in the previous exercise.

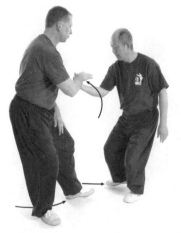

Start the exercise using the same techniques as in the first exercise. This time step into your partner's central door to close the distance for attack. Your partner will need to step away from your attack while simultaneously performing a yang or yin coiling action. Upon neutralizing the attack they will counterattack while stepping into your central door.

Continue to practice this exercise until you and your partner are able to neutralize and counterattack while stepping in a continuous motion. The next stage is to practice this exercise with your eyes closed. Once you have practiced this exercise to proficiency, you will change the hands to the left hand and repeat the procedures for the opposite side.

Tips to Avoid Common Errors. Common errors associated with the single hand exercise relate to the neutralization. When performing your coiling action, you must remember to keep your elbow alive. This means the elbow must move for an effective neutralization. Additionally, you must turn your body when neutralizing the attack. The arm must move with the body. Yin coiling must include a bowing of the chest such that the attack will be led away from your body. These movements should be emphasized while in the stationary position first. Finally, one must learn to stay attached to the partner throughout the entire exercise.

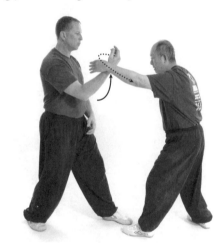

Once you and your partner have become proficient training opposite sides, practice listening and following training while you attach the hands on the same side. Practice this for both sides in both the stationary and stepping positions then close the eyes and repeat the exercise. Due to the repetitive nature of the exercise, we will not describe it in full detail here.

2. Double Hand (Shuang Shou, 雙手)

The next exercises involve using both hands with your partner. This simulates more of a pushing hands concept and is more realistic when encountering an opponent.

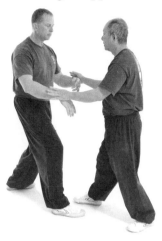

To practice this exercise, you and your partner should stand in the mountain climbing stance (deng shan bu, 登山步) with the right leg forward. Join hands at the wrists.

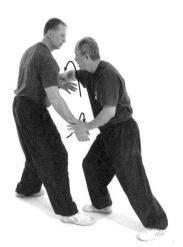

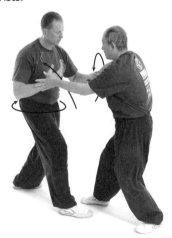

Next, either you or your partner will use either hand to attack the other. As one person attacks the other, it is the responsibility of the opposite person to recognize the incoming force, follow it, and use the yin or yang coiling movement to neutralize it. Once the attack is neutralized, that person will then follow with a counterattack.

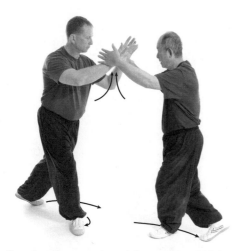

Practice the exercise while stepping. While stepping, the counterattack may also include a sealing action by one or both the attacking hands.

You and your partner will continue to practice this exercise until it becomes continuous and natural to follow the incoming force and redirect it for counterattacking. Finally, you will practice this exercise while keeping the eyes closed.

Tips to Avoid Common Errors. Common errors related to the double hand listening and following exercises are similar to the single hand errors. It is necessary to keep the elbow alive and moving in unison with your body when you are neutralizing the incoming force. From the defensive side of the exercise, you will need to pay more attention to your wardoff (peng, 掤) postures in order to avoid having your arms sealed against your body. This especially becomes prevalent when stepping. Additionally, you will need to pay attention to maintaining a safe distance while stepping for defense and closing the distance, or entering the central door, for attack.

3.6 Controlling Jing Training

Controlling jing is act of controlling the joint, or joints, of an opponent. While alternating between substantial and unsubstantial movements, you will neutralize your opponent's attack and control their joints. Of the two types of na jing, these exercises will focus on enhancing the skills of following, listening, and adhering. You will learn to stick to your opponent like a sheet of flypaper. These exercises are practiced while stationary and moving using both single hand and double hands. You will learn to control your opponent's wrists and elbows.

1. Single Hand (Dan Shou, 單手)

To practice this skill, begin in the stationary position. Stand facing each other with either the right legs or left legs forward. Your left hand may be placed out to the left side of your body, over your lower dan tian, or up by your opposite shoulder.

Place your right hand on your partner's left wrist and apply push (an, 按) to seal your partner's hand into their body. Your partner will apply wardoff jing (peng jing, 掤勁) and twist your body while coiling their hand over or under yours in an attempt to gain control over your wrist. You can use either a yang or yin coiling action. Once they have control, they can attempt to seal your hand into your body.

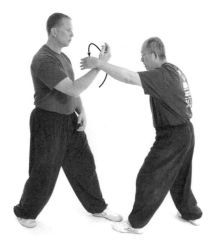 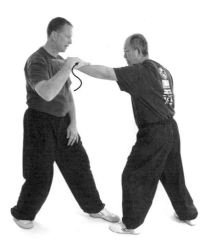

You then repeat the action of wardoff (peng, 掤) and coiling over or under their hand to once again control their wrist and seal their hand back into their body.

Practice this movement back and forth until it is smooth and continuous. Once you are both comfortable, you will each increase your effort in staying in control of your opponent's wrist.

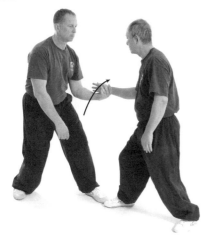

Next, change legs and practice the same exercise using your left hand and your opponent's right hand.

You will then switch back to the right leg forward and practice the exercise using your right hand and your partner's left hand. Follow this with switching back to the left leg forward and use your left hand with your partner's right hand.

The next stage of the single hand controlling jing training is to practice it while stepping. To do this, you and your partner will begin by facing each other and placing the right leg forward. With your right hand on your partner's left wrist, step into the central door while controlling their wrist. They in turn step back while applying wardoff jing (peng jing, 掤勁) and coiling around your wrist in a yin or yang direction in an attempt to gain control of your wrist joint. Your partner then returns the action by stepping into the central door while controlling your wrist. Practice this exchange back and forth then swap the forward leg to the left leg and repeat the exercise using the opposite hands. Finally, repeat the exercise while using the hands on the same side with the right leg forward followed by the left leg forward. Each time you both will increase your efforts at avoiding being controlled.

The next stage of controlling jing is to practice the control of your partner's elbow. Generally, this can be used as an attempt to seal the elbow into the body for uprooting the opponent.

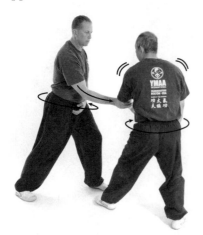

To begin this exercise, stand facing your partner with either the right or left leg forward. Place your right hand on your partner's left elbow and begin to push into their centerline. They will apply wardoff jing (peng jing, 掤勁) and coil their arm in either a yin or yang motion in order to place their hand on top of your right elbow.

They then apply push and attempt to seal your elbow into your body. Apply wardoff jing (peng jing, 掤勁) and coil around their arm using a yin or yang movement then return the pushing action into their elbow. Repeat this exercise back and forth until it is smooth and continuous. Follow this by switching the forward leg and repeating the exercise using the opposite hands. Then change the hands while keeping that leg forward and repeat the exercise for that side. Finally, switch to the opposite leg forward and finish the exercise by repeating the action with the opposite hands.

Tips to Avoid Common Errors. Common errors related to this exercise are similar to the previous exercise. The first is wardoff jing (peng jing, 掤勁) that must be applied when attacked. In order to perform the coiling technique properly one must keep the elbow alive. This means you will need to move your elbow around to allow the wrist to coil over the partner's wrist. Finally, be sure to keep your body and arm moving as one unit. Remember that the waist is the driver of the action. Twisting it back and forth will help you with coiling around the incoming force.

2. Double Hand (Shuang Shou, 雙手)

The next stage of training controlling jing is to practice the exercise using both hands. This training will provide you with more of the pushing hands atmosphere. Once again you will practice attacking the wrists and elbows while in stationary and stepping positions.

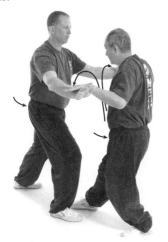 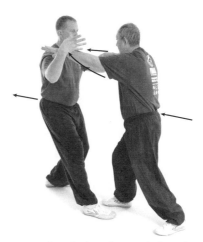

To begin the stationary training, stand facing your partner with right legs forward. Attach both your left and right hand to your partner's wrists then attempt to seal their hands into their body. You may choose to attack one side or both at the same time. Your partner applies wardoff (peng, 掤) and coils around your hands using either a yin or yang action. They then return the attack toward your body.

They also may choose to attack one of both sides. You will apply wardoff (peng, 掤), coil around their hands, and repeat the exercise.

The next exercise is to practice controlling the wrists with both hands while stepping. Face your partner in the mountain climbing stance (deng shan bu, 登山步) with the right legs forward.

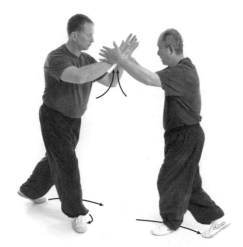

Repeat this exercise back and forth until you are both able to apply the coiling action in a yin or yang motion comfortably and smoothly.

The next exercise is controlling both elbows while in a stationary position.

Place your hands on your partner's wrists. Step forward into the central door while attempting to seal your partner's hands into their body. Your partner must step back to prevent your attempt at closing the distance, simultaneously applying wardoff (peng, 掤) and coiling around your hands to gain control of your wrists. Your partner will then step forward while attempting to seal your wrists into your body. You must step back, apply wardoff (peng, 掤), and coil around their wrists in order to avoid being sealed.

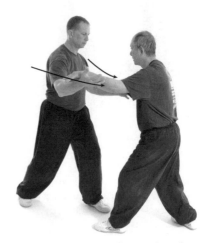

Your partner will apply wardoff (peng, 掤) and coil their arm or arms in a yin or yang fashion in order to gain back control and counterattack your movement by attempting

Face your partner with right legs forward. Place your hands on your partner's wrists. This time you slide either one or both your hands up to your partner's elbows in an attempt to seal their arms into their body.

to seal your arms into your body. Practice this exercise until the movements are smooth and comfortable. Once you have accomplished this, you and your partner should then practice attacking and neutralizing at the same time.

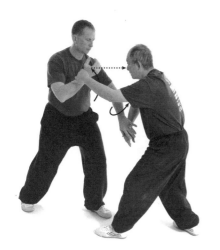

One person may be attacking one side and neutralizing the other.

In this exercise you and your partner will emphasize listening to both the insubstantial and substantial energy simultaneously. Practice this motion back and forth until you are both able to control the movements smoothly and continuously back and forth.

For the final exercise in this section, you will practice controlling both elbows while stepping. To do so, you and your partner will face each other with right legs forward.

Place your hands on your partner's wrists. Step forward to move into the central door while sliding your hands up into your partner's elbows in an attempt to seal the arms into your partner's body. Your partner will step back, apply wardoff (peng, 掤) and coil the arm or arms attacked using either a yin or yang action. Once they have gained control, your partner will then step forward while they attempt to seal your arms into your body. Repeat the exercise back and forth until you are both able to perform the movements smoothly and continuously. Finally, you and your partner should practice this exercise by attacking one side while neutralizing the other. Step back and forth while performing this exercise. Practice this until you are both able to do so effortlessly.

Tips to Avoid Common Errors. There are common errors to watch for within this training. Improper application of the use of peng energy, or lack thereof all together when defending against the incoming force, is common for beginners. This becomes more evident when training on the elbows. You also will have to focus on the use of both hands while attacking, neutralizing, and using the combination of both actions simultaneously. While stepping, you will need to focus on maintaining the central door while in defense and attempting to close the door while in offense.

3.7 Borrowing Jing

Borrowing jing is known as the ability to sense an opponent's attacking jing and borrow the energy before they manifest it. This is also called "striking the oppressive jing" (da men jing, 打悶勁). If the action was too late to sense the attack, borrowing jing may also be used at the end of the opponent's attacking jing. In this case the jing is expressed in between the end of the opponent's attack and the retreat of the attack. This is known as "striking the returning jing" (da hui jing, 打回勁). In both occasions you are finding the wuji state of occurrence and acting upon it. This requires a high sense of awareness between you and your opponent. Wǔ, Cheng-Qing (武澄清) wrote,

> When the opponent's jing is just coming and not yet emitted, I immediately strike. This is called "strike the oppressive jing"; when the opponent's jing has already come, and I have already been waiting, once (the opponent's jing has) reached my body, I strike immediately. When the opponent's power has entered the emptiness and is going to change (his) jing, I follow (his retreating) and strike, this is called "strike the returning jing." Experience the above (key words) and ponder carefully, (soon it will) follow (your) wish and reach the enlightenment naturally.[4]
>
> 人勁方來，未能發出，我即打去，此謂〝打悶勁〞；人勁已來，我早靜待，著身便打去，人已落空，欲將換勁，我隨之打去，此謂〝打回勁〞。由此體驗，留心揣摩，自然從心所欲階及神明矣。

From this statement you will see the necessity to train attaching, listening, following, and connecting jings. You will need to be able to sense the incoming attack and react immediately. You should also be able to sense the change from the attack to return and be able to counterattack at this time. In both cases you are using bumping (kao, 靠) jing patterns to control your opponent.

> What is called question and answer in taijiquan is to investigate the opponent's movement and calmness. Its goal is to listen (for) the direction and heavy center (i.e., the origin of the root) of his jing. This means to probe the opponent's situation. It is what is called to gauge the opponent. Before the opponent and I engage in battle, I should use the calmness to wait for the labor without any formed opinion (i.e., guessing). The opponent does not move, I do not move. The opponent slightly moves, I move first. The most precious moment is the instant of mutual exchange between the opponent and I, when (if I) know the opponent's insubstantial and substantial, I can deal with it. All of these (possibilities) are originated from (the) feeling of listening jing, insubstantial and substantial, question and answer, and gauging the opponent. The practitioner should pay attention to put all the effort in these.[5]

太極拳之所謂問答，即問其動靜。目的在聽其勁之方向與重心，即偵
察敵情之意，所謂量敵也。彼我在未進行攻擊以前，吾應以靜待動，
以逸待勞，毫無成見。彼未動，我不動，彼微動，我先動。貴在彼我
相交一動之間，即知其虛實而應付之。此均由於感覺。聽勁、虛實、
問答、量敵而來。學者應注意致力焉。

Master Wu, Gong-Zao (吳公藻) further explains the necessity of gauging your opponent. One must stay calm and listen to your opponent's intentions. Through constant training you will gain the experience of foresight. When the opponent doesn't move you will remain still. Once the opponent's physical manifestation of intent is initiated, you have already moved, thus intercepting the incoming force. This is considered a very high level of awareness or borrowing jing.

As you can imagine there are many ways to train borrowing jing. In the next section we will offer a few methods to develop your borrowing jing essence. Keep in mind this is considered a higher level of training, and in order to reach this level you must be consistent in your training. For each of the following exercises it is best to begin slowly. Once you have consistently been able to perform the exercise smoothly, you then will increase the speed.

The first exercise trains the method of "striking the oppressive jing."

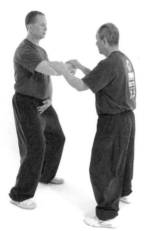

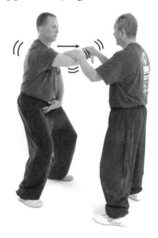

Stand facing your partner in a ma bu position. Place your right arm out in front of you with the arm parallel to the ground at approximately chest height. Your partner will place their hands on your wrist and elbow.

Your partner chooses when to apply the push (an, 按) movement on you. You in turn listen for this movement and apply wardoff (peng, 掤) prior to the actual action occurring. After a few repetitions switch to the left hand and have your partner apply push (an, 按) to that arm.

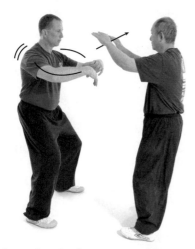

For the final stage of this exercise you will close your eyes while practicing the exercise using one arm, then the other arm, and finally both arms. You may also practice this while on bricks to enhance the training.

The next exercise is striking the returning jing.

Next, place both arms up and have your partner apply push (an, 按) to both arms. In this example the partner places their hands on your wrists to apply their action.

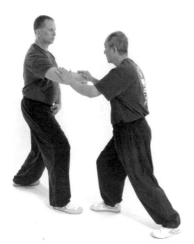

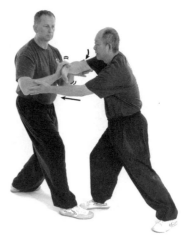

Face each other with the right legs forward. Your right arm is parallel to the ground at shoulder height. Your opponent places their hands on your wrist and elbow and applies push (an, 按) while you yield and horizontally neutralize the attack.

To neutralize, shift your weight back, twist your body to your right, and allow your partner's hand to move to your right. As you coil your hand over your partner's wrist, you begin to pluck their wrist while your partner ends their attack and is beginning to retreat.

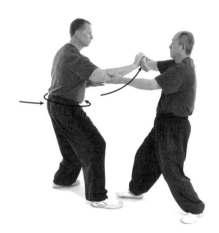

From this position you change to pressing your partner's wrist back toward them which increases the force back into the direction they originated.

Continue to practice this action until you are able to perform it smoothly on your partner. Then, change position so your left leg is forward and practice the same exercise for your left arm. The final stage of this exercise is to practice them all with your eyes closed. To get even deeper in your training, repeat all the exercises while standing on bricks, followed by closing your eyes while on bricks.

Tips to Avoid Common Errors. For both striking the oppressive jing and returning jing you must have the proper timing. Signs of improper timing are either a large bumping or a double weighted feeling on the oppressive side and a jerking action on the returning side. To avoid this, build on your listening skills. It is important to begin slowly while applying the techniques. As you become more proficient, build up the speed of attacking and applying the borrowing jing.

References

1. "練拳不練功，到老一場空。"

2. "一舉動，週身俱要輕靈，尤須貫穿。太極拳論，張三豐。" Dr. Yang, Jwing-Ming, *Tai Chi Secrets of the Ancient Masters* (Wolfeboro, NH: YMAA Publication Center, 1999), 1.

3. "其根在腳，發於腿，主宰於腰，形於手指。由腳而腿而腰，總須完整一氣。太極拳論，張三豐。" Dr. Yang, Jwing-Ming, *Tai Chi Secrets of the Ancient Masters,* 3.

4. Dr. Yang, Jwing-Ming, *Tai Chi Secrets of the Wǔ and Li Style* (太極拳武、李氏先哲祕要) (Wolfeboro, NH: YMAA Publication Center, 2001), 27.

5. Dr. Yang, Jwing-Ming, *Tai Chi Secrets of the Wu Style* (太極拳吳氏先哲祕要) (Wolfeboro, NH: YMAA Publication Center, 2002), 37.

Chapter 4: Single/Double Pushing Hands Training

4.1 Introduction

In the following section we introduce both the single and double pushing hands exercises. There are solo exercises and two-person exercises, and these actions are done while in the stationary position, rocking, and stepping.

4.2 Stationary Single Pushing Hands

The first exercises are the single stationary pushing hands exercises. Practice in the ma bu position followed by the rocking position. Initially practice solo then practice with a partner. Each time you are performing the neutralizations solo, imagine an individual is attempting to find your center by attaching to your wrist and applying a force in toward you. When practicing the neutralizations with a partner, the individual who is pushing will initially apply their force in toward the center of the partner's body. This allows the opposing person the chance to choose which neutralization to apply. As each individual advances in skill, the incoming force may be applied in different directions. The practice of leading the neutralization in the direction of the incoming force develops listening jing (ting jing, 聽勁) skills. In order to properly apply each technique it is important to first train your body movements correctly before applying them to a partner.

We will introduce four possible neutralizations. For each of these neutralizations, the first movement necessary for neutralizing the incoming force is to create the wardoff (peng, 掤) posture throughout your body. This structure has been emphasized throughout numerous taiji classics. To create the posture, you must round out the back while closing the chest and arcing the arms. The tailbone is slightly tucked under while the head is in the upright position. For the push hands movement, the arm your opponent is attacking will be initially in a horizontal position approximately chest height. When performed correctly, your pectoral muscle should remain fairly loose. This posture is often the most neglected initial movement and necessary for you to evade your partner's attempt to find your center and thus control you.

1. Horizontal Neutralization (Shui Ping Hua, 水平化)

The first neutralization in single push hands training is the horizontal neutralization.

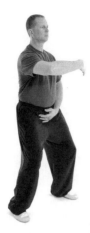

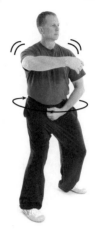

To begin this exercise, stand in the ma bu position with your right arm approximately chest height and parallel to the ground. The right wrist is vertically aligned with your sternum.

To initiate the neutralization, create the wardoff (peng, 掤) posture as described earlier. Inhale and twist your body to the right until the right wrist is vertically aligned with your right shoulder. Now the incoming force is considered to be neutralized.

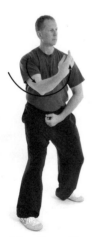

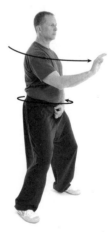

Lower the right elbow. Your palm will be facing you. Turn over your palm so it faces away from you. Begin to exhale as you twist your body back to the forward facing position.

The right arm will begin to extend while your right hand begins to apply the push (an, 按) action.

Your chest opens as this movement is occurring. Once your hand returns to the original position, raise the right elbow and repeat the neutralization as before. Continue to practice this movement back and forth until you are able to perform the exercise continuously with the proper body movements. Once you are able to do so, practice this exercise using the left hand.

Now that you are comfortable with the movement, practice the movement with your training partner. Stand facing each other in the ma bu stance.

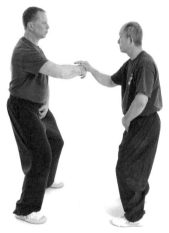

Bring your right arm up to the initial position. Your partner places their hand on your wrist and elbow.

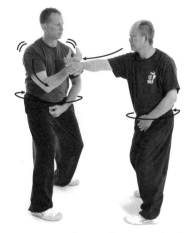

Your partner applies push to your body. You neutralize the force by applying peng, by twisting your body to your right and horizontally neutralizing the action. Next, you lower your elbow.

Your partner in turn uses the same actions of peng, horizontally neutralizing and pushing back toward you. Repeat this continuous action back and forth until you both are able to perform it smoothly and continuously, then repeat the exercise for the left arm.

The next step is to practice this neutralization using the rocking motion. Although it will be described with a partner here, you may practice this without a partner first if you wish.

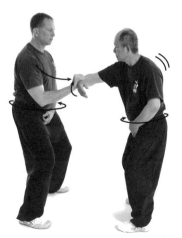

Rotate your palm so that it is placed on your partner's wrist and apply push back toward their body.

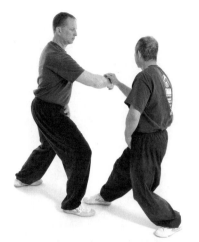

Begin this exercise by standing in the mountain climbing stance (deng shan bu, 登山步) with your right leg forward. Place your right arm in front of your body parallel to the ground just as you did in the stationary exercise. Your partner places their hand on your wrist.

Your opponent applies push to your wrist. In this situation you apply two actions, yielding and neutralizing. First create the wardoff (peng, 掤) structure. Inhale and begin to twist the waist to the right while shifting your weight back into the four-six stance (si liu bu, 四六步). You can now see the yielding motion is the shifting of the weight while the neutralization is the twisting of your body. The end of this neutralization occurs when the right hand is vertically aligned with your right shoulder and you are in the four-six stance (si liu bu, 四六步).

Once the hand reaches the original position, return to the original posture and repeat the exercise. Continue to practice this exercise until you are able to perform the actions continuously with the proper body movements. This exercise should also be practiced using the left leg forward.

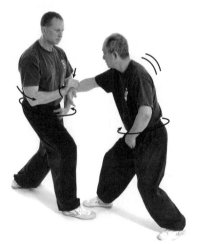

To return to the original position, lower the right elbow while rotating the right palm over to face away from you. Begin to exhale while simultaneously shifting your weight forward into the mountain climbing stance (deng shan bu, 登山步) and twisting the waist back to the facing forward position. The right arm will extend, with the hand once again applying the push (an, 按) or pushing action and your chest will begin to open up.

2. Downward Neutralization (Xia Hua, 下化)

The next exercises are known as downward neutralization. This neutralization occurs on the same side as the horizontal neutralization.

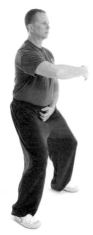

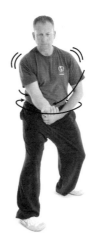

To begin this exercise, stand in ma bu with your right hand approximately chest height, arm parallel to the ground.

Inhale while creating the wardoff (peng, 掤) posture. Twist your body to the right and rotate your right forearm, turning the right hand palm up to create a coiling action to roll over an incoming force. This action will cause your elbow to lower itself toward your body. The end of the neutralization occurs with the right hand now approximately waist height and vertically aligned with the right shoulder. The right elbow will be approximately one fist's distance from your body and the right arm will be parallel to the ground.

Once your hand has reached the original position, raise the right elbow till the right arm is parallel to the ground. Rotate the palm to face back toward you and repeat the downward neutralization. Continue this exercise until you are able to do the exercise continuously with the proper body movements. Once you have completed this exercise, repeat the action using the left hand.

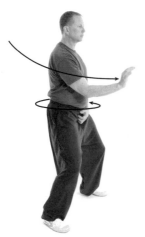

Rotate the hand, palm facing away from your body, and begin to twist back to the forward facing position while exhaling. The chest will now open while you apply an with the right hand.

Next, practice downward neutralization, in the ma bu position, with your partner.

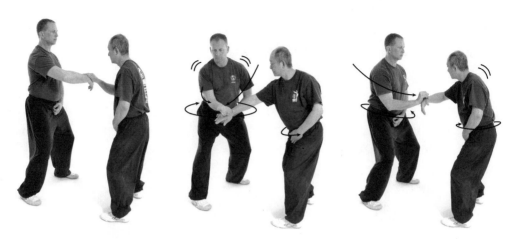

Downward neutralization with a partner.

The actions are the same as solo except that now you are able to feel your partner's incoming force; neutralize it, and return the pushing action into your partner so they may also neutralize the incoming force.

The next step is to practice downward neutralization while rocking. You may want to practice this exercise solo to familiarize yourself with the synchronization of the neutralization and rocking. Here we will describe the exercise with a partner.

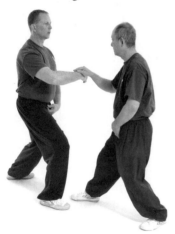

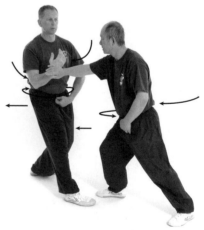

To begin, stand in the mountain climbing stance (deng shan bu, 登山步) with the right leg forward. Your right arm should be parallel to the ground with the right hand approximately chest height.

As your partner applies push, inhale while first creating your wardoff (peng, 掤) posture. Twist the waist to the right while shifting the weight back into the four-six stance (si liu bu, 四六步). The right elbow drops down toward your body while the right hand coils over, palm facing up.

This is the end of the neutralization. From this position inhale, rotate the palm away from your body, and begin to shift the weight forward into the mountain climbing stance (deng shan bu, 登山步) while opening the chest and applying the an action with the right hand. Once the right hand reaches the original starting position, return to the original posture and repeat the downward neutralization exercise. Continue to practice the exercise until you can move continuously with the proper body movements throughout the exercise. Once you have completed this exercise, practice the movements with the opposite leg forward.

3. Upward Neutralization (Shang Hua, 上化)

The next neutralization is known as upward neutralization. This neutralization occurs on the opposite side as the previous two neutralizations.

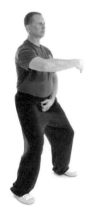 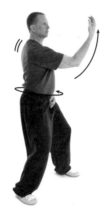 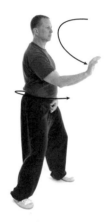

Stand in the ma bu stance with your right arm parallel to the ground, approximately chest height.	Inhale while creating the wardoff (peng, 掤) posture throughout your body. Twist your body to the left and raise your right hand up to approximately face height. The wrist will remain facing you.	Begin to twist your body back to the right. As your hand passes through your midsagittal plane, rotate your right wrist so the palm now faces forward. Lower the right hand, begin to exhale, and apply your push (an, 按) technique.

Once the hand reaches the original starting point, rotate the palm back toward you and reset your posture for the next neutralization. Continue these movements until you are able to complete the actions continuously with the proper body movements. Once you are able to do this, change hands and practice this exercise with the left hand.

Next, repeat this exercise with a partner.

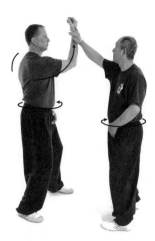

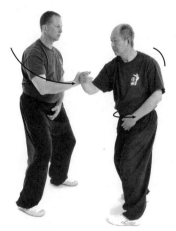

Your partner applies push on your wrist directly into your centerline while you apply peng. Twist to your left, raising your hand upward then twisting back to the right.

Passing the vertical centerline between you and your partner, rotate your palm and lower your hand to attach to your partner's wrist. Apply push to your partner's wrist and they will repeat the same actions of upward neutralization.

Repeat these movements back and forth until you both are able to do so using the proper movements in a continuous manner.

Rocking. The next step for this exercise is to practice it while rocking. You may elect to practice this action solo first to get used to the movements while rocking. Here we will describe the exercise with a partner.

To begin, face your partner while standing in the mountain climbing stance (deng shan bu, 登山步) with the right leg forward. The right wrist is in front of the chest with the right arm parallel to the ground. Your partner places their right hand on your wrist and applies push toward your centerline.

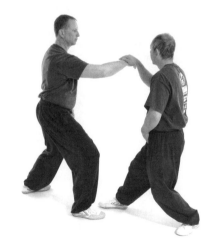

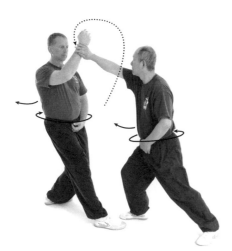

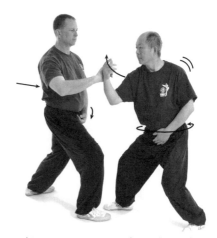

Inhale, apply peng, and begin to shift your weight back into the four-six position (si liu bu, 四六步). Simultaneously twist your body to the left while raising the right hand to approximately face height just as you have while practicing solo. Reaching the four-six stance (si liu bu, 四六步) position, twist back to the left. Keep your right palm facing you until passing the vertical centerline between you and your partner.

From this position, rotate the palm and lower the hand to approximately chest height. Place your hand on your partner's wrist and apply push to their centerline while you exhale and rock forward into your mountain climbing stance (deng shan bu, 登山步). Your partner will then neutralize your incoming force using the same technique of upward neutralization.

Continue this exercise until you are both able to perform the actions continuously using the proper movements. Once you have accomplished this task, place the left feet forward and repeat the exercise using the left hand.

4. Sideways Neutralization (Ce Hua, 側化)

The final exercises in the single pushing hands training are sideways neutralization. This neutralization is similar to the upward neutralization. It assumes the incoming force continues past the normal range.

Stationary.

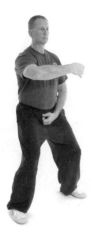

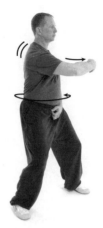

Begin sideway neutralization training in ma bu stance with the right wrist in front of your chest. The right arm will be parallel to the ground.

Begin to inhale and twist your waist to the left. Your right hand will remain chest height until it reaches your left shoulder.

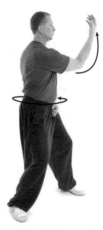

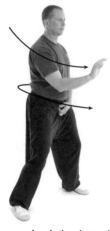

Once it has reached this position begin to raise it up to face height.

Next twist your body back to the right. Keep the palm facing you until it passes the midsagittal plane then turn the palm away from your body and lower the hand to approximately chest height. Begin to exhale and apply your push (an, 按) technique with the right hand.

Stationary. The next stage is to practice this exercise with your partner.

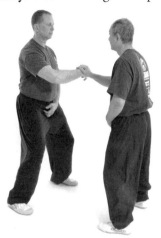

Stand in the ma bu position with your partner facing you. Your partner places their
hand on your wrist and pushes into your
centerline.

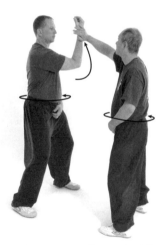
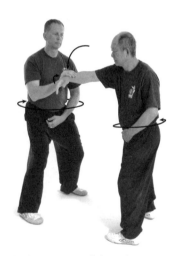

Repeat the actions you performed while solo. First twist left with the arm parallel to the
ground, then raise your right hand up approximately to face level. Twist your body back to the
right and, crossing the vertical plane between the two of you, rotate your palm and place your
hand on their wrist to apply push toward their centerline.

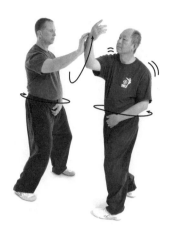

Your partner twists their body to the left and begins the sideways neutralization.

Once your right hand reaches the original starting position, reset your body posture so you may repeat the exercise. Continue to practice this exercise until you are able to perform the proper actions smoothly. Once you are able to do this correctly, practice the same movements using the left hand.

Rocking. The final sideways neutralization exercise is to practice while rocking. As with all these exercises, you may first practice them by yourself to get familiar with the movements, then with your partner. Here we will describe the actions with a partner.

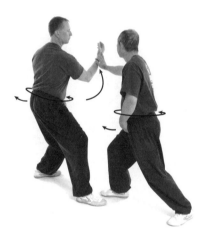
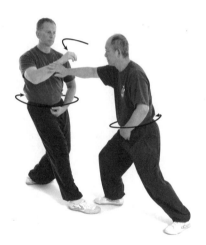

To start this exercise, face your partner and step into the mountain climbing stance (deng shan bu, 登山步), both of you with your right legs forward. Place your right wrist in front of your chest with the right arm parallel to the ground. Your partner places their hand on your wrist. As they begin to apply an into your centerline, you begin to inhale, apply peng, rock aft into the four-six stance (si liu bu, 四六步), and twist your waist to the left. The right hand initially remains on a horizontal path until it is vertically aligned with the left shoulder. From this position, raise the right hand to approximately face height. Twist your body back to the right, keeping the palm facing you until it passes the vertical plane between the two of you then rotate the palm away from your body and place your hand on your partner's wrist.

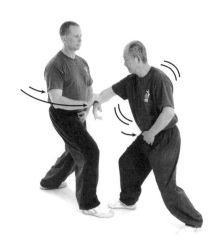

Begin to exhale and apply the push (an, 按) technique toward their centerline while shifting the weight forward into the mountain climbing stance (deng shan bu, 登山步). At this point your partner begins to use the sideways neutralization followed by returning an back toward you.

Continue to practice this exercise back and forth until you both are able to perform the proper body movements effortlessly. Once you are able to do so, place the left leg forward and repeat this exercise for the left hand.

4.3 Moving Single Pushing Hands

4.3.1 Basic Step Training (Ji Ben Zou Bu Lian Xi, 基本走步練習)

This stage of single pushing hands includes stepping while neutralizing and attacking. After all, in a real situation you are not going to stand in place while your opponent strikes you; nor is your opponent going to simply stand there, allowing you to neutralize their attack and then counterattack them. This type of exercise begins to train you in the deeper meaning behind five of the Thirteen Postures or actions of taijiquan. You will learn to change the location of the wuji point while stepping and in doing so apply less effort in redirecting your opponent's attack. You will also discover the importance of remaining centered while changing your location in reference to your opponent. Before you train the moving section of this training, you will need to understand a few concepts and practice these actions with a partner to grasp a deeper understanding of this knowledge.

The first concept is the definition of a central door (zhong men, 中門) and empty door (kong men, 空門).

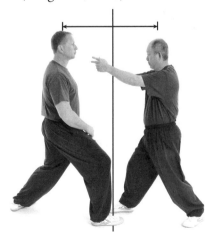

When two individuals are facing each other, there is a certain distance between them. This distance or space between the two opponents is known as the central door (zhong men, 中門). The aggressor will want to close the distance and occupy the central door.

Central door (zhong men, 中門).

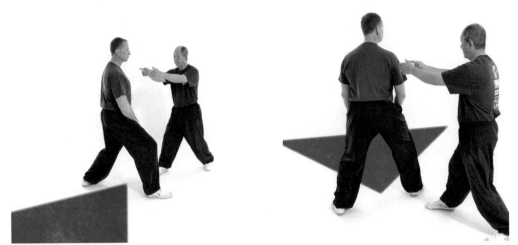

Empty doors (kong men, 空門) are located on angles either in front of the opponent or behind the opponent.

The empty door (kong men, 空門) is the area that provides an opponent a chance for attack or take down without being attacked from the opponent's opposite side. It can be thought of as an area to which you are able to walk through the opponent. Empty doors are located on angles either in front of the opponent or behind the opponent. They are designed for attacking and uprooting your opponent. The main concept is to avoid allowing your opponent to enter the central door and empty door for attack. You can defend this area by stepping away from your opponent and re-entering the central door for your counterattack. This counterattack should be done on an angle so as to enter your opponent's empty door

Once these concepts are in place, you need to practice the techniques of listening, following, adhering, and attaching as applied to the central and empty door.

4.3.2 Stepping (Zuo Bu, 走步)

The first stage of this training is the solo stepping stage. In this exercise you learn how to focus the mind through the ground and increase your feeling through the feet while stepping.

In order to do this stepping exercise properly, it is suggested you practice while using a shoe with little to no padding, or you may practice barefoot. It is also recommended to practice this exercise outside either on grass or on a sandy beach. This training conditions the joints of the ankle, knee, and hips. In addition to strengthening the joints, you become more aware of the uneven ground upon which you are stepping. All this training helps the mind and body communicate with your surrounding area.

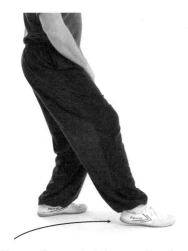

To step forward, slide your foot forward, without lifting the toes away from the ground, while maintaining a slightly squatted position.

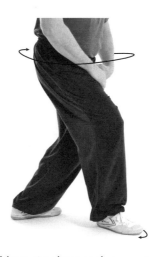

Next, simultaneously turn your body and forward foot laterally. This stance is a transition stance known as zou pan bu.

From this position, slide the aft foot forward. Your body should be level throughout the entire movement. Do not bounce up and down. This allows your legs to change the angle of bending over uneven ground and allow your upper body to remain relatively stable throughout the movement.

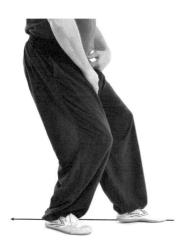

To step backward, draw the body back by shifting the weight to the back leg. The body should assume a wardoff (peng, 掤) posture. As this occurs, the forward foot slides back to the aft position.

You will notice that your forward foot will be turned outward. Simply turn it back to its original forward facing position once you have shifted your weight slightly aft. Continue to step forward and back over various surroundings while focusing on sliding the feet rather than lifting them up. Once you are comfortable with this, you may also choose to change the direction of stepping from linear to angled stepping. Stepping on an angle is performed by placing the sliding foot on a diagonal to the direction of your original path. If you are familiar with the art of baguazhuang you may also continue further with walking in the bagua circle stepping. This will help you with changing the angle of attacking as well as yielding and neutralizing during pushing hands training. The final stage is stepping with eyes closed. This allow you to increase the feeling in your feet to a deeper level.

4.3.3 Sense of Distance (Ju Gan, 距感)

The next stage of this training is to practice the stepping in a linear direction with a partner. The training increases the range of focus from the foot to the object you are attached to. In this exercise, you attach to your partner by touching each other's wrist. Remember, you are actually sensing your opponent's body and not just the hand. If they are stepping correctly, the increased pressure you may feel from the attack is coming from the opponent's entire body and not just the hand. The main concept of this exercise is not to lose contact with your partner and not to cause a bump or a situation where you are double weighted, all while keeping in motion. Double weighting occurs when there is no distinction between insubstantial and substantial forces. This can occur on either a single side or double side. Taiji classics say, "(When the opponent presses) sideward (or) downward, then follow. (When there is) double weighting (i.e., heaviness or mutual resistance), then there is stagnation."[1]

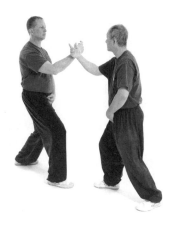

Sense of distance training.

To practice this exercise, face your partner with the right legs forward. Extend your right arm out and touch your partner's wrist with the palms facing inward. The opposite hand will be placed out to the side for balance. Next, begin to step forward, occasionally pausing in between steps, while attempting to close the distance between the two of you. Your goal is to attempt to enter the central door while your partner's goal is to keep you from entering the central door. After you have reached the end of your practice area, reverse the roles and allow your partner to attack while you retreat. Continue to step to the opposite end of the practice area then repeat the exercise. Once you are both comfortable with your listening, following, attaching, and adhering jing, practice this exercise by moving back and forth, exchanging your attack and retreat in a more free-style manner. This training increases your jing skills because you now have to listen more carefully to your partner. Initially, you may find a situation where you both may wish to attack and this will cause a bumping or double weighted situation. Continue to practice this exercise until you and your partner are able to remain attached to each other's wrist while stepping forward and backward.

The next stage is to perform the same actions while attaching to both hands.

Next, have your partner place their hands on your wrists. In each case the hands on top are simulating a controlling position. Continue to practice this stage back and forth until the movements are smooth and continuous.

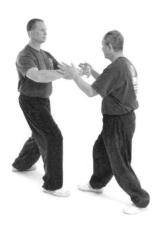

Place your hands on top of your partner's wrists and practice moving back and forth for attack and retreat.

For the next stage, continue to practice the actions of stepping back and forth while changing from double hands to single hands and back to double hands.

Eventually, increase the level of training. Close your eyes while performing the exercise.

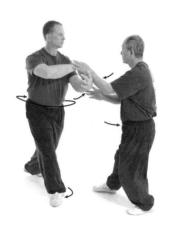

Begin stepping back and forth using the double hands method. As you step forward or backward, use your yin-yang circling techniques to move either hand across to your partner's opposite hand.

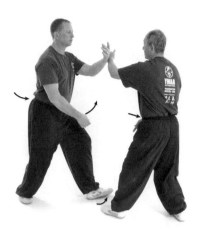 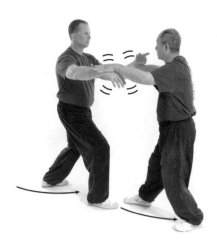

In this situation, it is important to allow the opposite hand to remain attached to your partner in the transition. You may also transition back to double hands using the same yin-yang circling motion.

4.3.4 Sense of Angling (Jiao Du Gan, 角度感)

In this set of exercises, you and your opponent focus on entering into the empty door. As previously explained, the empty door is the area that represents an open doorway that you would be able to walk through. Your goal is to be able to enter your opponent's empty door for attacking the sky window or the ground wicket. The sky window is the area located from the solar plexus to the head. The ground wicket is the area from the solar plexus to the feet.

Due to the endless combinations of stepping and exchanging of hands, we will not explain in detail the actions of stepping and attacking or stepping and withdrawing. The main concept here is that you and your partner are stepping on an angle, either to the left or right, to enter the empty door while coiling over the other person's hand with your own hand.

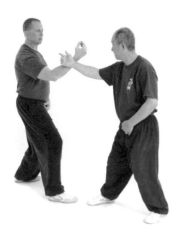

Stand facing your partner with the right legs forward. Extend your right hand and touch each other's wrist.

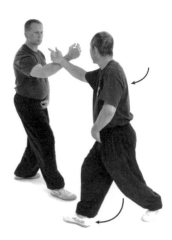

As either one of you step toward the opposite person's empty door, that person will react by stepping on an angle, either left or right, to defend their empty door.

Keep in mind that you may switch hands as well as use both hands whenever attacking or neutralizing. However, do not be too concerned with the actions of the hands at this stage. At this stage of the training, it is more important to focus on the distancing and angling techniques of stepping. Continue this exercise until both you and your partner are comfortable stepping in on the angle for attack as well as stepping away on angles for neutralizing an incoming force.

4.3.5 Basic Self Yin-Yang Neutralization Practice
(Ji Ben Yin-Yang Hua Zi Wo Lian Xi, 基本陰 / 陽化自我練習)

The next set of exercises focuses on the coiling, circling, and spiraling techniques necessary to neutralize an incoming force. You will train both the yang and yin sides of neutralizing while in the stationary and rocking positions.

Yang Coiling Neutralization—Solo

Stationary.

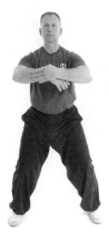

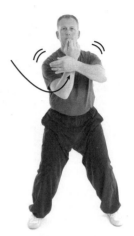

Stand in the ma bu stance. Hold your arms out in front, approximately chest height, Select either the left or right hand and place it on the outside of the opposite wrist.

Inhale while circling the elbow of the inside hand down. The chest will close and you will coil the inside hand over the opposite wrist.

The fingers of the coiling hand should be relaxed and covering the whole area. Continue to practice this until you are comfortable with the movements. Next, shift your weight as you coil one hand over the opposite wrist.

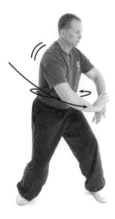

Exhale while settling the hand over the wrist. The ending position is where one hand is touching the wrist of the other, sealing the arm down.

Rocking.

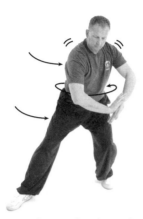 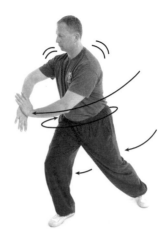

Place the right leg forward and stand with equal weight on both legs. Place one hand in front of the wrist of the opposite hand and begin to coil the hand in the aft position over the top of the opposite hand while inhaling and closing the chest. The elbow of the coiling hand will circle down while the hand begins its path over the top of the opposite hand's wrist. As the hand coils over the wrist, exhale, twist the body, and shift your weight either forward into a mountain climbing stance (deng shan bu, 登山步) or back into a four-six stance (si liu bu, 四六步).

End in either stance with the coiling hand sealing the opposite arm downward. From this position, begin to coil the inside hand over the opposite hand while twisting the waist and inhaling. As the hand coils over the top, continue to twist the waist while exhaling and shifting the weight, ending once again in either mountain climbing stance (deng shan bu, 登山步) or four-six stance (si liu bu, 四六步).

The coiling hand will again seal the opposite arm down and your body will be twisted in that direction. Continue to practice this exercise until you are able to perform the yang coil on either side of your body. This should also be able to be demonstrated in a forward or backward position. Once you are comfortable performing this exercise you should change position and practice the same method with the left leg forward.

Yin Neutralization Training—Solo

Stationary. The next sets of exercises use the yin coiling method of self yin-yang neutralization. Perform these exercises while in the ma bu position as well as shifting stances between mountain climbing stance (deng shan bu, 登山步) and the four-six stance (si liu bu, 四六步).

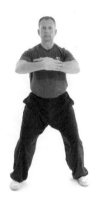 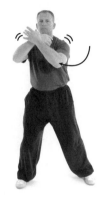 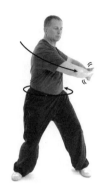

Stand in the ma bu stance and place your arms at chest height with one hand touching the wrist of the opposite hand.	Begin to inhale while coiling your inside hand under and around then over your outside wrist.	From this position, pluck the outside wrist while twisting your waist to the side of the plucking hand.

To change to the opposite side, reset to the original forward facing position while rotating the palms back facing you. You then repeat the action for the opposite hand and twist to the opposite side. Practice this exercise for both sides until you are able to perform the movements properly and smoothly throughout.

Rocking. Next, perform these exercises while shifting your weight between the mountain climbing stance (deng shan bu, 登山步) and the four-six stance (si liu bu, 四六步).

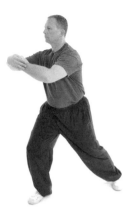
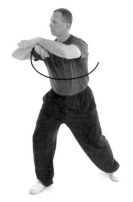
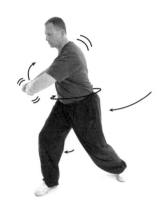

To begin, stand in the mountain climbing stance (deng shan bu, 登山步) and place your arms up at chest height with one hand attached to the opposite wrist.

Inhale while coiling the inside hand around the opposite arm. As your hand coils over the opposite arm, the opposite hand simultaneously plucks it while shifting back into the four-six stance (si liu bu, 四六步).

From this position you may elect to perform the yin neutralization from there and end in the mountain climbing stance (deng shan bu, 登山步), or you may reset yourself to the original position and practice the exercise again.

Once you are comfortable performing this exercise, place the opposite foot forward and practice the movements once again. Continue to practice these exercises until you are able to do so comfortably and smoothly with proper body movements. We should note that even though we have illustrated the movements to one side you may yin coil and move in either direction.

4.4 Stationary Double Pushing Hands

The following exercises involve the use of both hands. These exercises are for the most part the same as those we have described in the stationary single push hands section. Before beginning this exercise it is necessary to train the opposite hand in an exercise known as elbow neutralization. It is written,

> (When using) zhou (i.e., elbow) to strike, (it) is as a cow bowing its head. Blossom the flowers (with) linking attack as (you) wish. This (technique) is used with close range when cai (i.e., pluck) is applied (on you). (If it is) used at the long range, (you will) earn the shame by the opponent. (When) the opponent uses cai (i.e., pluck) to seal me, (I) apply (elbow stroke) following the (opponent's) posture. Pointing the elbow to the ribs' tendons, (the opponent's) life will be rested (i.e., ended). (When) using the elbow (to strike), the most fearful (technique) against (you) is the posture of playing guitar. When encountered, turn the body (to protect) my throat.[2]

肘打好似牛低頭，開花連環任自由。

此是近取一採手，遠距用之氣人羞。

對方封采隨勢用，肘指肋脅一命休。

用肘最怕琵琶勢，遇之轉身我咽喉。

In tai chi pushing hands the primary attack is with the palm. However you and your opponent are in close range and as such one must also be aware of the opponents elbow. In his writing Master Li, Yi-Yu discusses this use of Zhou. It has both offensive and defensive purposes which are only for short range. If used in a long range you will be in vain. Zhou is used against a person applying Cai and when done so you follow your opponent to attack the rib area. Alternatively you may find yourself in a situation whereby your opponent is attempting to control your elbow and you will use your peng energy in combination with circling the elbows to neutralize the attack. The following exercises will assist you and your partner in the use of Zhou neutralization.

4.4.1 Elbow Neutralization

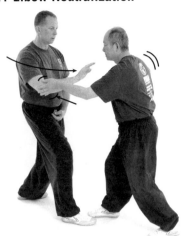

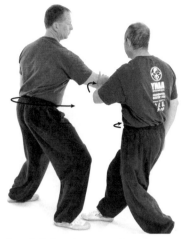

Face your partner. Raise your right arm and attempt to push or touch your partner's solar plexus. Your partner places their left hand on your elbow, thumb on top. As you reach for your partner's solar plexus, they will twist their body to the right and pluck (cai, 採) your elbow to the right.

As their left hand passes the center vertical plane between the both of you, they turn the left hand over so the fingers now rest on top of your right elbow. They are attempting to seal your arm into your body by applying push (an, 按) on your arm.

Continue this exercise until you are both able to execute it in a smooth and continuous action, then exchange the movements so you are also able to practice applying the plucking/sealing technique to your partner. Practice this exercise until you are both comfortable applying this technique. It should be done in a continuous flow using the proper movements before attempting to move on to the double push hands exercises.

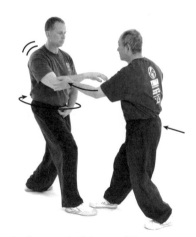

You apply the wardoff (peng, 掤) posture and twist your body back to the right in order to avoid their push and return to the original position. Reaching the original position, you once again attempt to touch their solar plexus.

1. Horizontal Neutralization (Shui Ping Hua, 水平化)

The first exercise in double push hands training is the horizontal neutralization exercise. You will train these exercises with your partner while standing in the ma bu position as well as rocking. As always, you may first practice the movements solo to get used to the coordination of the hands with the rocking of the body. Here we will only describe the partner exercises.

Stationary.

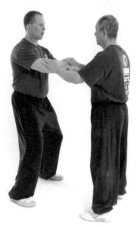

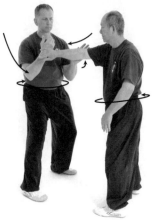

Stand in ma bu and face your partner. Your arm should be horizontal at about chest height. Your partner places their hands on your wrist and elbow in preparation to apply an to your centerline.

Your partner applies push (an, 按). You apply peng and twist your body to the right while performing the same movements of the single hand horizontal neutralization with your right hand. As you twist to the right, extend your left hand and attach it to your partner's right elbow, palm facing up. Continue to twist to the right and simultaneously lower the right elbow while turning the left palm over your partner's elbow to neutralize your partner's force.

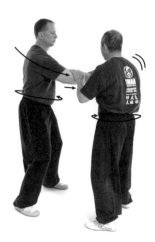

After you have neutralized your partner's force, apply the an technique back toward your partner's centerline by twisting your body to the left while both palms turn over attaching to your partners wrist and elbow.

Continue to practice the neutralization back and forth until you are both able to do it smoothly while using the proper body movements. Change to the left hand horizontal neutralization and practice the same movements for the opposite side.

Rocking. The next exercise is the double push hands horizontal neutralization with your partner while rocking. To begin this exercise, you and your partner will face each other with the right leg forward. Place your right hand out in front of your body approximately chest height while your partner attaches to your wrist and elbow with their hands.

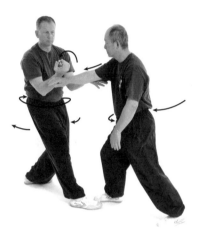

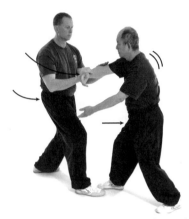

While your partner applies push (an, 按) into your centerline, inhale, apply peng and begin to shift your weight back into the four-six stance (si liu bu, 四六步), yielding to the incoming force. As you shift back, twist your body to the right and perform the actions of the double hand neutralization previously described. The left hand, palm up, will reach forward, intercepting your partner's right elbow while the right hand neutralizes the incoming force to the right. Once your right hand is vertically aligned with your right shoulder, lower the right elbow and rotate the right hand so the palm faces away from the body.

The left hand will rotate over and attach to your partner's right elbow. Twist the body back toward the left and apply your push (an, 按) technique into your partner's centerline while exhaling.

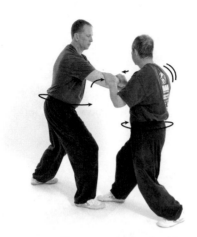

Your partner will now apply the double hand horizontal neutralization then return their attack.

Continue this exercise until you are both able to perform the proper body movements continuously back and forth. Once this has been accomplished, place the left foot forward and practice the same neutralization with the left hand in front of the chest.

2. Downward Neutralization (Xia Hua, 下化)

The next set of exercises are the downward neutralization exercises. This will be practiced first while in the stationary position followed by the rocking position with your partner. You may also elect to practice this solo to become familiar with the movements. Here we will only describe the two-person interactions.

Stationary.

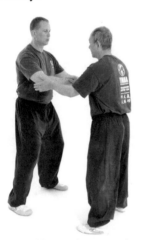

Stand in ma bu. Your right arm is horizontal, approximately chest height. Your left hand is also at about chest height. Your partner places their hands on your wrist and elbow. Your left hand should be placed by your chest area in preparation for intercepting the elbow of your opponent.

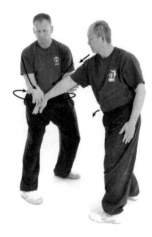

As your partner applies an into your centerline, inhale, assume the wardoff (peng, 掤) posture and twist your body to the right while performing the downward neutralization just as you have done in the single push hands exercise. The left hand will now extend forward to intercept your partner's elbow and apply the plucking (cai, 採) technique. Once your right hand is aligned vertically with the right shoulder, the neutralization is complete.

Continue to practice your neutralizations back and forth until the movements are continuous with the proper body actions. Once you have completed this, change to the left hands and complete the downward neutralization for the opposite side.

Rotate your left hand over your partner's right elbow while turning your right hand over to face your partner's right wrist. Your partner at this point will recognize the neutralization along with the need to no longer attack. You will both twist back to the forward facing position where you will now apply your pushing (an, 按) technique into your partner's centerline. They will in turn apply the downward neutralization then return to applying the an technique to you once you both return to facing each other.

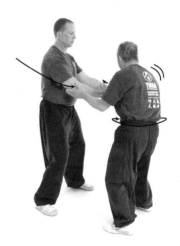

Rocking. The next method of practicing the two-person downward neutralization is in the rocking position.

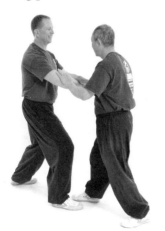

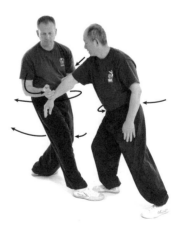

To begin this neutralization, you and your partner will stand in the mountain climbing stance (deng shan bu, 登山步), right legs forward. Place your right arm at chest height parallel to the ground. The left hand will once again be placed in front of your chest aligned with the left shoulder. Your partner will place their hands on your wrist and elbow and apply an into your centerline.

Inhale while constructing the wardoff (peng, 掤) posture. Shift the weight back into the four-six stance (si liu bu, 四六步) while twisting the body to the right and applying the downward neutralization technique previously described.

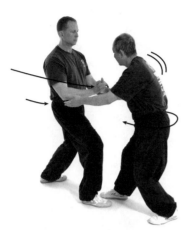

As you are completing the technique, twist back to the forward facing position, rotate both the left and right hands over, placing them on your partner's wrist and elbow. Shift back into the mountain climbing stance (deng shan bu, 登山步) while applying your push (an, 按) technique back into your partner's centerline.

Your partner will now perform the downward neutralization technique then return the an movement back toward you to repeat the exercise. Once you have reached your original starting position, repeat the downward neutralization. Continue to practice this exercise back and forth until you are both able to perform the movements smoothly using the proper body actions. Once you are comfortable doing this, you and your partner should place the left leg forward and complete the neutralization for the left side.

3. Upward Neutralization (Shang Hua, 上化)

The next exercise is the two-person upward neutralization. These exercises are done in the ma bu position followed by the rocking position.

Stationary.

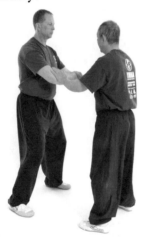

Begin in the ma bu stance. Place your right hand out in front of your body approximately chest height parallel to the ground. The left hand will be placed out in front of your chest, vertically aligned with your left shoulder. Your partner will place their hands on your wrist and elbow.

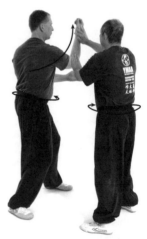

As your partner applies an, inhale and begin the neutralization with the wardoff (peng, 掤) posture. Twist the body to the left while applying the upward neutralization described in the single pushing hands section.

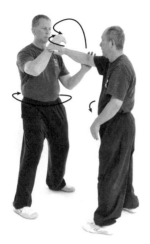

From this position, attach to your partners' wrist and elbow and apply the push (an, 按) technique toward their centerline. They follow this action with the upward neutralization and return to applying an toward you in order to keep a continuous flow back and forth. Continue to practice this exercise until you both are able to perform the correct movements throughout the maneuver. Once your body is comfortable doing this exercise with the right hand, switch to the left hand and repeat the exercise.

Rocking. Next, you practice the two-person upward neutralization while rocking.

Once you have neutralized your partner's attack, twist your body to the right. The left hand extends, palm facing up, and intercepts your partner's right elbow. As you continue twisting to the right, the left hand will turn over, palm facing down, while the right hand rotates palm facing out.

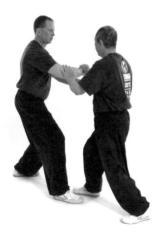

To begin this exercise, face each other with the right leg forward. Place your right hand out in front of the chest with your left hand out by the chest area. Your partner places their hands on your wrist and elbow.

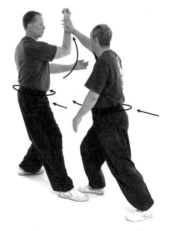

When they apply an to your centerline, you inhale and begin your neutralization with the wardoff (peng, 掤) posture. Simultaneously twist the body to the left while shifting to the four-six stance (si liu bu, 四六步).

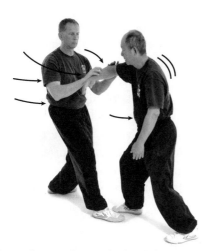
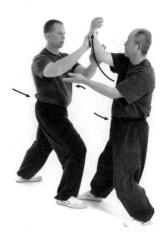

Once the attack is neutralized, begin to twist your body back to the right. Your left hand intercepts the partner's right elbow with the palm facing up. As your right hand passes the vertical plane between both of you, turn your palms over in preparation for returning the pushing action. Begin to exhale and shift the weight into the mountain climbing stance (deng shan bu, 登山步) while applying the an technique to your partner's centerline.

Repeat this action continuously until you are able to do this exercise smoothly with the proper body movements. Once this is complete, change the forward leg to the left one and practice the exercise using the left hand.

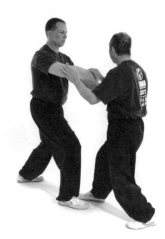

Your partner follows this action with practicing the upward neutralization and repeating the an movement back to you.

4. Sideways Neutralization (Ce Hua, 側化)

The next neutralization is the two-person double push hands sideways neutralization. This neutralization follows the same methods applied by the single push hands except you are now adding the left hand to neutralize your partner's elbow.

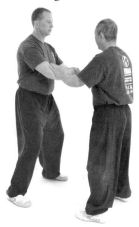

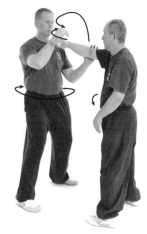

Begin in the ma bu stance. Place your right hand in front of your chest and the left hand by the chest approximately on the same side as your left shoulder. Your partner will place their hands on your wrist and elbow then apply an into your center-line.

Inhale and begin the neutralization with your wardoff (peng, 掤) posture. Twist the body to the left and apply the sideways neutralization you practiced in the single push hands section. The left hand, palm up, intercepts your partner's elbow as your body is twisting back to the right. Both palms turn over as your right hand passes the vertical plane between you and your partner then you begin to exhale, open your chest, place your hands on your partner's wrist and elbow, and apply your push (an, 按) technique into their centerline.

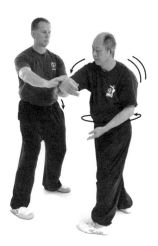

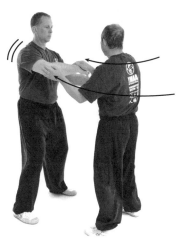

They then perform the sideways neutralization followed by returning the an technique back to you.

Repeat the exercise until you are both able to execute the neutralization smoothly using the correct body postures. Once this has been completed, you should practice the same methods described for the opposite hand.

Rocking. The next exercise is the sideways neutralization while in the rocking position. To do this, stand in the mountain climbing stance (deng shan bu, 登山步), right leg forward, with your right hand placed out in front of your chest. The left hand will be either by your left hip or near the right armpit. To initiate the neutralization, inhale while applying the wardoff (peng, 掤) posture then shift the weight back into the four-six stance (si liu bu, 四六步) while twisting the body to the left. The right hand will once again perform the same action of sideways neutralizing that was done in the single push hands section. Once you have begun twisting back to the right, your left hand, palm up, will extend out in front of your body to intercept your partner's elbow. As the right hand passes your centerline, turn both palms over in preparation for returning your push (an, 按) technique. Next, exhale and shift your weight forward while applying push (an, 按). Once you have reached back to the original position, repeat the neutralization. Continue to practice these movements until they become smooth with the correct body postures. After you have completed this task, you should place the left foot forward and repeat the neutralization for the opposite hand.

5. Elbow Following Neutralization (Zhou Shun Hua, 肘順化)

The next exercise is known as the elbow neutralization or repelling neutralization exercise. This exercise focuses on neutralizing the incoming force on your elbow first. You and your partner will practice this movement while both in the stationary and rocking position. As with all the neutralizations, you may practice them solo first then with a partner if you want to get used to the feeling of the movements. Here we will only describe the movements with a partner.

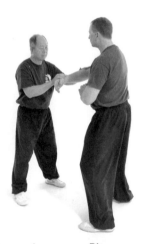

Stand in the ma bu stance. Place your right hand out in front of your chest and the left hand out in front of your chest area vertically aligned with your left shoulder. Your partner will place their hands on your wrist and elbow and apply the push (an, 按) technique toward your centerline. Inhale and assume your wardoff (peng, 掤) posture.

Stationary.

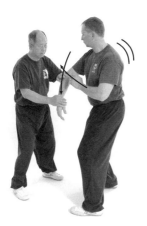 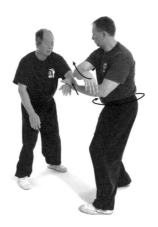 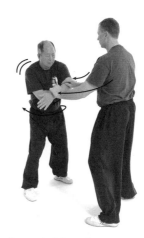

Twist your body to the left while moving your right arm down toward your left hip. As your right elbow crosses your centerline, slide the left hand, palm out, under and outside of your right elbow.

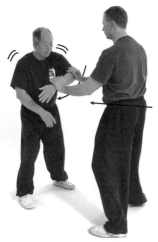 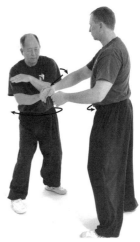

Attach your left hand to your partner's wrist, twist your body back to the right, and draw your right arm back to the right, placing both your hands on your partner's left arm. From this position you apply push (an, 按) to your partner's left arm while they perform the neutralization.

The one difference you will notice here is that it will be done on the left arm. Once they have applied the neutralization to you they will apply push (an, 按) to you and it will be repeated for the right arm. Repeat the neutralization back and forth until you are both able to perform the technique correctly with the proper body movements. Switch to having your left arm up initially and repeat the exercise, neutralizing to the opposite side.

Rocking. The next exercise is to practice the two-person neutralization while rocking. To practice, face each other with right legs forward. Place your right hand out in front of your chest with the left one approximately chest height and vertically aligned with your left shoulder. Your partner will place their hands on your wrist and elbow and apply push (an, 按) to your centerline.

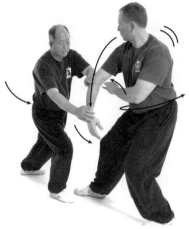

Inhale and begin the neutralization with your wardoff (peng, 掤) posture. Twist your body to the left, moving your right arm down toward the left hip. This will be done while you shift back into the four-six stance (si liu bu, 四六步) position.

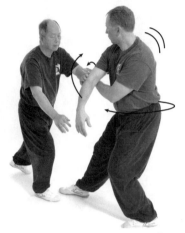

As your right elbow passes your centerline, slide the left hand, palm facing out, under and outside the right elbow, attaching to your partner's left wrist area.

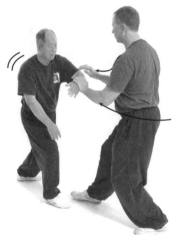

Twist the body back to the right while drawing the right arm back to the right, attaching to your partner's left elbow.

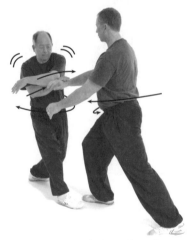

From this position, exhale and apply your push (an, 按) technique to their centerline as you shift back to the mountain climbing stance (deng shan bu, 登山步) position. Your partner, in turn, applies the same neutralization using their left arm, simultaneously shifting aft while applying peng and twisting to the right, intercepting your wrist with their right hand.

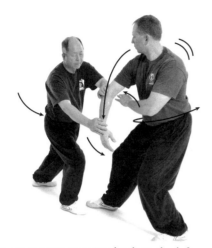

Next, your partner twists back to the left while placing their left hand on your right wrist and applies push (an, 按) to your centerline while shifting forward. From this position you will once again repeat your neutralization.

Continue this exercise until you are both able to perform the neutralization smoothly with the correct body movements. Once this is complete, switch legs (left forward) and repeat the exercise for the opposite side.

6. Elbow Smearing Neutralizing (Zhou Mo Hua, 肘抹化)

The final exercise for the double push hands section is known as the neutralizing elbow or smearing neutralization. This action also focuses first on neutralizing the elbow and will be done both in the ma bu stationary position as well as the rocking forward and aft position. You will notice that, unlike the previous exercise, you remain on the same side. In other words, after you complete the neutralization you return to the original position. If you start with your right arm, after you complete the neutralization your opponent's hand will be on your right arm again, and vice versa.

Stationary. Begin in the ma bu stance. Place your right hand out in front of your chest and the left hand by your chest area approximately aligned vertically with your left shoulder. Your partner will place their hands on your wrist and elbow and apply push (an, 按) to your centerline.

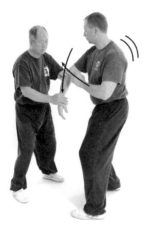

Inhale and apply the wardoff (peng, 掤) posture. Twist your body to the left, allowing the right hand to move down toward the left hip. As the right elbow approaches the central vertical plane between you both, slide your left hand, palm down, over your right elbow and up to your partner's left wrist.

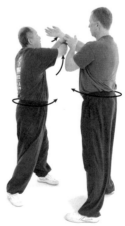

Begin to twist your body back to the right while circling the right arm counterclockwise. Your right hand rotates, palm up, and reaches for your partner's left elbow.

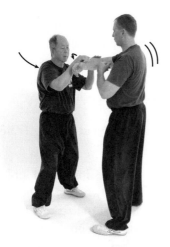

Continue this exercise until you are able to practice the neutralization continuously and smoothly. Switch positions and allow your partner to train the neutralization before moving to the rocking position.

Rocking. Next you will perform the two-person double hands neutralization while rocking. To begin this exercise, face each other with the right legs forward. Place your right hand out in front of the chest with your left hand approximately chest height and vertically aligned with your left shoulder.

Your partner follows you with their right hand intercepting your right arm from underneath and slides their left arm back. This neutralizes your counterattack and you both twist back to face each other. Your partner places their hands on your right wrist and elbow while you return back to your original position.

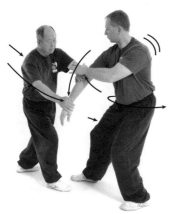

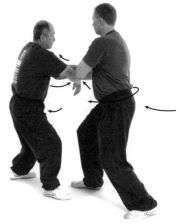

Your partner will place their hands on your wrist and elbow then apply an to your centerline. Initiate the neutralization by inhaling and applying your wardoff (peng, 掤) posture. Twist the body to the left, moving the right hand down toward your left hip while shifting your weight back into the four-six stance (si liu bu, 四六步). With the right elbow approaching the central vertical plane between you and your partner, slide your left hand up over your right elbow onto your partner's right wrist.

Twist back to the right while shifting forward into the mountain climbing stance (deng shan bu, 登山步) and circle your right arm, palm up, counterclockwise, reaching for your partner's right elbow. Your partner in turn follows your action and circles their right arm under your arms to neutralize your counterattack.

From this position they retract the left arm and you both return to your original positions with your partner applying an to your centerline and you neutralizing the attack. Practice this exercise until you are able to neutralize the attack continuously and smoothly then change positions so your partner may practice the neutralization as well.

4.5 Moving Double Pushing Hands

The next stage of training is to practice pushing hands while stepping linearly and on angles. Taijiquan consists of the Thirteen Postures or actions. Five of these are stepping actions, one of which is being centered. One should understand that being centered is not restricted to a stationary position. You must also be able to remain centered while stepping in any direction. You may have begun to realize you are using less energy to deflect or lead your opponent's attack to the wuji point. You may also be finding that the ever-changing wuji point reveals itself in a timelier manner and with less effort on your part. This is the path to the deeper levels of taijiquan training. When you engage an opponent in real situations, there are endless combinations of defense and attack and you have a myriad of choices in the direction necessary for proper yielding, neutralization, and counterattacking techniques.

4.6 Peng/Lü/Ji/An International Double Pushing Hands

The next exercise is an internationally known pushing hands routine that illustrates the use of wardoff (peng, 掤), rollback (lü, 摭), press (ji, 擠), and push (an, 按). This exercise will be practiced while stationary, rocking, stepping linearly, then changing angles while stepping.

Stationary. The first method of practicing wardoff (peng, 掤), rollback (lü, 攦), press (ji, 擠), and push (an, 按) will be in the stationary position.

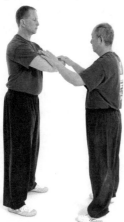

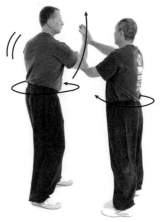

Begin in the ma bu stance. Place your arms at approximately chest height with the palms facing inward, assuming a ji posture. Your partner places their hands on both your elbows to control your joints.

Your partner begins to apply the push (an, 按) action on your arms in an attempt to seal your arms down into your body, exposing your sky window (upper region of the torso and head), for attack. You neutralize the incoming force by first applying wardoff (peng, 掤), then continuing with upward neutralizing.

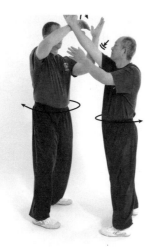

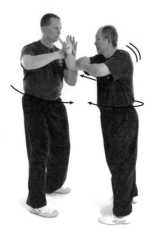

The neutralization can be executed in either direction. As your arms cross the central vertical plane between the two of you, you start applying rollback (lü, 攦) in an attempt to lock their elbow.

Your partner's next movement is to evade this lock by rotating their forearm palm up while dropping their elbow on the arm to which your lock is being applied. Of course, doing this exposes them to being sealed at the elbow so they follow this action by sliding their hand toward the opposite elbow and applying press (ji, 擠).

Next, reverse your roles and repeat this action back and forth until you are both comfortable applying each of the actions described. Be sure to apply the neutralization equally toward either direction.

Rocking. The next method of practicing this exercise is with rocking.

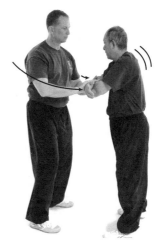

Your partner now assumes the press (ji, 擠) posture while you assume the push (an, 按) posture with your hands placed on their elbows.

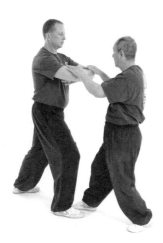

To begin this exercise, stand facing your partner with the right legs forward. Once again you place your arms out in front of the body at approximately chest height and your partner places their hands on their elbows.

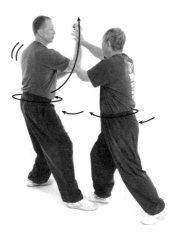

Your partner applies their push (an, 按) technique while simultaneously rocking forward. You apply the wardoff (peng, 掤) posture followed by upward neutralizing and rollback (lü, 攦) while rocking back.

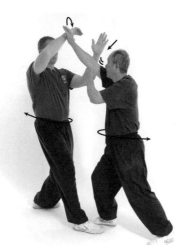

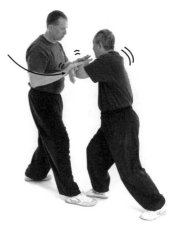

Remember, this neutralization can and should be applied in either direction. Twist your body and place your arm on your partner's elbow while plucking their wrist in an attempt to lock their elbow.

Your partner rotates their forearm and drops their elbow to avoid the lock then slides their hand into the pocket of the opposite elbow and applies squeeze or press (ji, 擠) toward you.

You now have your hands on their elbows and begin to apply the push (an, 按) technique while rocking forward. Your partner then applies wardoff (peng, 掤), upward neutralizing, followed by rollback (lü, 捋) while rocking back. As they attempt to lock your elbow, you neutralize the elbow and apply press (ji, 擠) back into them. This brings the exercise back to the beginning. Continue to practice these movements back and forth until you both are able to apply the techniques smoothly with the correct body movements. Be sure to apply the neutralization in both directions. You should also switch leg positions and practice the same exercise.

Stepping. The next method of practicing this exercise is while stepping in a linear motion.

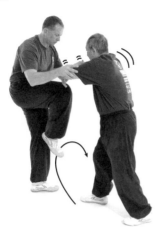

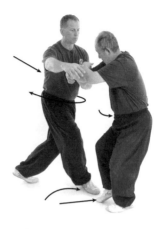

To begin this exercise, you and your partner face each other with the right legs forward. Next you begin to apply the push (an, 按) technique to your partner's elbow joints in an attempt to seal their arms down into their body. While this is occurring, lift your forward leg, simulating a potential kick to the opponent's vital areas.

Place your foot next to the outside of your partner's foot while continuing to move forward.

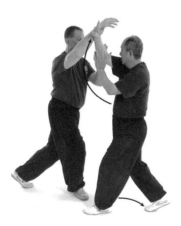

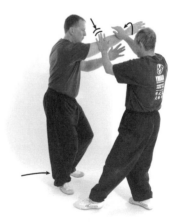

Your partner responds to your actions by twisting their body, shifting their weight backward, and applying wardoff (peng, 掤) followed by upward neutralization.

Your partner then steps back while applying the rollback (lü, 擟) technique in an attempt to lock your elbow. You step forward while rotating the forearm and dropping the elbow.

From this position you both switch roles. Continue to practice this exercise while stepping forward and backward in a linear direction until you and your partner are able to perform the actions continuously using the correct body movements. Be sure to neutralize your partner in both directions.

Change Angling (Bian Jiao Du, 變角度)

The final stage of this wardoff (peng, 掤), rollback (lü, 攦), press (ji, 擠), and push (an, 按) training is to add the skill of stepping on angles. The stepping expands on the options you have for defensive and offensive moves.

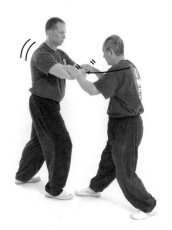

Next, step forward while sliding your hand into the opposite elbow to perform press (ji, 擠). Your opponent steps back, ending with their hands on your elbows.

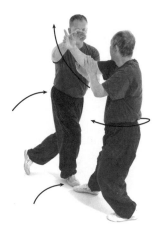

To begin, you and your partner face each other with right legs forward. Next, you begin to perform the push (an, 按) technique while stepping forward. Your partner will step back on an angle and neutralize.

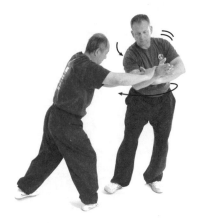

As your partner begins to lock your elbow, rotate your forearm and lower your elbow. Slide the other hand into the inside crease of your opposite elbow and begin to apply press (ji, 擠) while stepping on an angle into your partner's empty door.

Continue to practice this exercise back and forth until you are both able to execute the actions smoothly and without interruption. Be sure to neutralize your partner's incoming force in both directions.

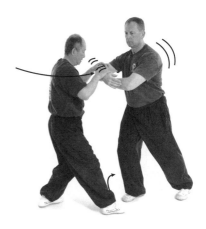

You and your partner are now in opposite roles and you can now repeat the exercise in the opposite direction.

Tips to Avoid Common Errors.

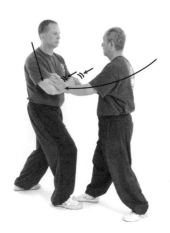

The wardoff (peng, 掤) posture that follows the initial attack by the partner must be applied when your partner applies his push (an, 按) technique; otherwise, you are allowing your partner to seal your arms into your body.

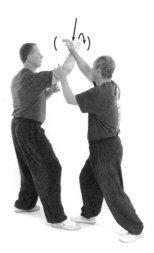

You also need to watch for turning your hand too early when changing into the rollback (lü, 擟) movement. Be sure to keep your palm facing you until you turn your body enough for the arm to pass the centerline between you and your partner. Otherwise your partner will have an easier avenue to seal your arm into your body.

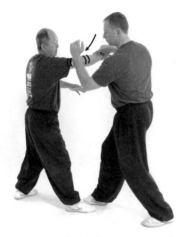
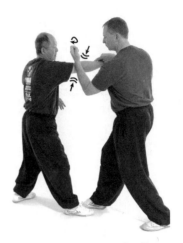

During the rollback (lü, 掘) movement, do not use your hand to intercept your partner's elbow, use your arm. Place your arm so that your radius and ulna are parallel to your partner's triceps tendon. Then twist the forearm to grind the tendon while you shift your weight back, performing rollback (lü, 掘).

Stepping in a linear direction can be tricky for this exercise. Practice slowly and if necessary, practice the stepping sequence first then add the hands. Take three steps forward when you attack. Take two steps backward when you retreat. The initial step is followed by the rollback (lü, 掘) movement so you are shifting your weight from front to back while your opponent takes their second step forward, neutralizing your rollback (lü, 掘) action. Finally, be careful to properly apply your wardoff (peng, 掤) posture in both directions when you step linearly or at an angle.

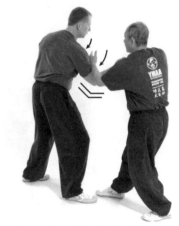

When neutralizing the rollback (lü, 掘) action on the elbow, drop the elbow while simultaneously applying wardoff (peng, 掤) and stepping up into your partner's central door.

References

1. 〝偏沉則隨，雙重則滯。〞 Dr. Yang, Jwing-Ming, *Tai Chi Secrets of the Wu Style* (太極拳 吳氏先哲祕要) (Wolfeboro, NH: YMAA Publication Center, 2002), 46.

2. Dr. Yang, Jwing-Ming, *Tai Chi Secrets of the Wǔ and Li Style* (太極拳武、李氏先哲祕要) (Wolfeboro, NH: YMAA Publication Center, 2001), 87.

Chapter 5: Taiji Rollback/Press Pushing Hands Training

5.1 Introduction

In the next section we address the movements of small rollback (xiao lü, 小攦), large rollback (da lü, 大攦), and press (ji, 擠). In taijiquan, there are two forms of rollback: large and small. Each one of these movements incorporates the use of wardoff (peng, 掤), yield (rang, 讓), lead (yin, 引), and neutralize (hua, 化) jing. The focus of these movements is to lead the opponent into emptiness. Once you have led the opponent into emptiness, you can return with a press (ji, 擠) or bump (kao, 靠) jing. Strategically speaking, the difference between small and large rollback is that small rollback (xiao lü, 小攦) utilizes small and quick movements that expose your opponent's cavities for striking. Large rollback involves larger movements designed more to pull your opponent's root, causing them to lose balance and providing you with the opportunity for further attack. Large rollback usually involves more stepping techniques than small rollback (xiao lü, 小攦).

Before reviewing the exercises of large and small rollback (xiao lü, 小攦) along with press (ji, 擠), we will introduce a few common training exercises designed to prepare you for the rollback and press.

1. Press Neutralization (Ji Hua, 擠化)

The first exercise introduces the neutralization of pressing. This may be practiced while standing in the ma bu position as well as facing each other with either leg forward. For our examples here we will describe the actions using the right leg forward.

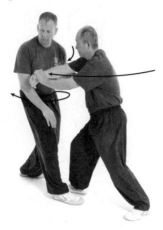

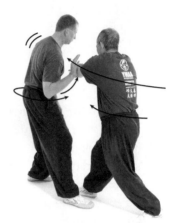

Your partner applies ji or press into your solar plexus. As you feel the incoming force being applied, apply wardoff (peng, 掤) while twisting your body and shifting it aft to neutralize the incoming force. If you neutralize the incoming force to the right, you will twist your body to the right while you apply wardoff (peng, 掤) and raise your left hand to meet the outside section of your partner's forearm.

If you neutralize to the left, twist your body to the left while applying wardoff (peng, 掤) and raise your right hand to intercept the outside section of your partner's forearm.

Next, allow your partner to neutralize your press into their solar plexus. Continue to practice this method of neutralization back and forth with your partner until you are both comfortable with neutralizing the incoming force. The neutralization should be smooth, with an emphasis on leading the incoming force into emptiness.

The next stage of practice is to neutralize using wardoff.

Also practice the neutralization using the left or right arm passing completely under both your partner's arms so it ends up across and outside of their arms (your right arm on the outside of your partner's right arm or your left arm outside of your partner's left arm). This movement prepares you to change sides. You and your partner should continue to practice these exercises until you both can do them smoothly and in a continuous motion, with proper body movements.

2. Elbow Neutralization 1 (Zhou Hua 1, 肘化－1)

The next exercise works on the neutralization of the elbow in the rollback training. This exercise builds on the wardoff (peng, 掤), rollback (lü, 攦), press (ji, 擠), and push (an, 按) training exercises.

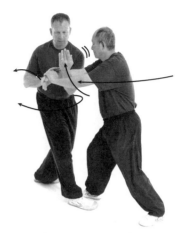

Your partner applies press toward your center. You use wardoff (peng, 掤) and twist the body to one side while moving the arm up in between the other person's arms.

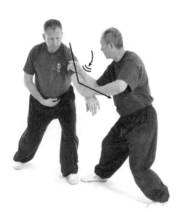

Face your partner with your left leg forward. Your partner has their right leg forward. To begin, allow your partner to pluck your left wrist while placing the right forearm just above the elbow joint.

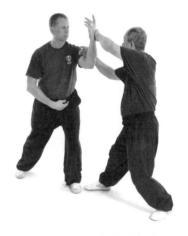

Your partner rotates their right forearm in order to grind the tendon of the elbow joint or attack the tianjing (TB-10) (天井) cavity. Once you feel the pressure being applied to your elbow joint, rotate your forearm, which allows the elbow to drop and neutralize the force.

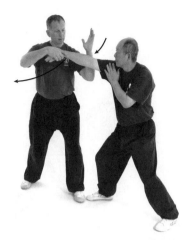

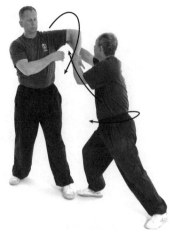

Next, apply wardoff (peng, 掤) energy with your left arm, twist the waist, and turn toward your partner. The right hand immediately reaches over your left arm and plucks your partner's right wrist in order to protect your face from attack. Your left forearm slides up above your partner's right elbow joint and you begin to apply the rollback force to your partner's arm.

Rotate your left forearm in an attempt to grind your partner's elbow joint. Your partner rotates their right forearm to drop the elbow and applies wardoff (peng, 掤). Next, your partner twists back toward you, reaches over their right arm, and intercepts your left wrist with their left hand.

This places you both at the beginning of the exercise and you can repeat the actions back and forth. Continue to practice this exercise back and forth until it is smooth and continuous. Change the position of your legs in order to practice this movement on the opposite arms.

3. Elbow Neutralization 2 (Zhou Hua 2, 肘化 2)

This last exercise is also designed for neutralizing the elbow. This situation simulates the case where you may attack an opponent's arm to apply your large rollback (da lü, 大 挒) technique and find their arm is bent so that it is not possible to lock the elbow. Rather than struggle to apply the technique, learn to attack with a different technique. This exercise gives you a second option to neutralize an attack on your elbow joint.

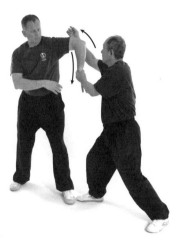

Stand side by side with your partner. Your partner begins to pluck your left wrist. Begin to bend your arm. Your partner slides their right arm up toward your elbow and they apply pressure just above and inside the elbow joint with their right forearm while plucking your left wrist.

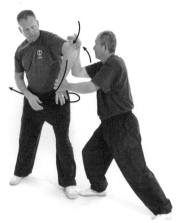

Your partner twists their body to the left while attempting to lock your arm and cause you to fall. As you feel the pressure applied to your elbow, you neutralize this by applying peng and scooping your arm down toward your hips.

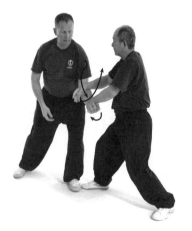

Twist your body to the left while you rotate your palm up and circle your elbow back toward your body, completing the neutralization of your partner's action.

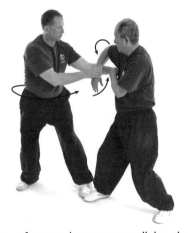

As your forearm becomes parallel to the ground, continue to twist back toward your partner and prepare to execute your rollback on them. Slide your left hand up toward your partner's right elbow while moving your right hand over your left arm and up to your partner's right wrist for plucking.

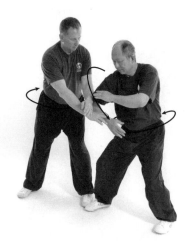 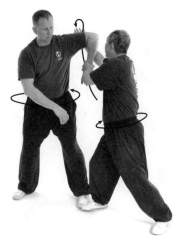

Your left arm now slides up under your partner's right elbow and you twist to the right once again in order to apply the technique to your opponent. As you execute your rollback technique to your partner, they now twist to their left while applying wardoff (peng, 掤) and redirecting your force.

Once your partner has neutralized your attack, they twist back toward you while sliding their right arm up to the back side of your left arm. With their left hand plucking your left wrist, they repeat the rollback technique on you.

From this position you may repeat the neutralization techniques back and forth. Continue to practice this exercise until you are both able to perform the technique smoothly. Finally, you both need to change legs and practice the technique for the opposite arms.

Tips to Avoid Common Errors. The common errors mainly occur during the neutralization of the elbow itself. In the first exercise, it is necessary to drop the elbow by rotating the palm and forearm upward. You must also be aware of not allowing the elbow to be sealed against your body when you neutralize the attack. In the second exercise the elbow is already bent in one direction, so you need to move the arm toward your body in order to redirect the incoming force. In both exercises the waist needs to be loose and alive in order to redirect the movements. You need to twist the body back toward your partner in order to gain control of their arm and apply the technique.

5.2 Small Rollback and Press

The first exercises in this section are the small rollback (xiao lü, 小擺) and press (ji, 擠) exercises. These exercises are not currently on the taiji pushing hands DVD series but are important to train.

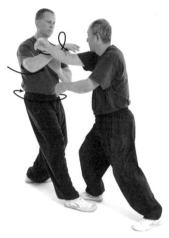

Face your partner with your right legs forward. Place your right wrist on the outside section of your partner's right wrist and begin to spiral over their arm toward their elbow in a clockwise motion.

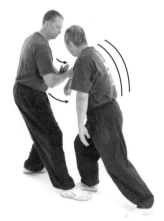

As you reach for your partner's elbow, rollback by shifting your weight aft and twisting your body to the left. Slide your left hand up to your right wrist and begin to press (ji, 擠) toward your partner's body.

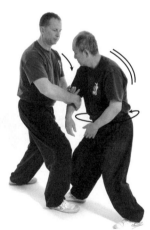

Your partner initially neutralizes this press by shifting their weight back, turning their body to the left and applying wardoff (peng, 掤) to your attack.

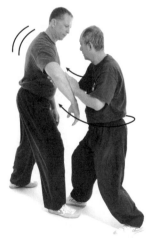

As they continue to shift their weight back, they spiral their right hand clockwise over your right arm until their hand is on the inside section of your right elbow.

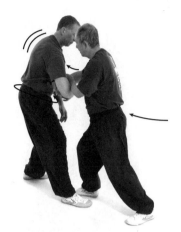

They then slide their left hand up to their right wrist and apply press (ji, 擠) to your body.

From this point you neutralize the attack by twisting your body to the left and applying wardoff (peng, 掤) to their incoming force. Your right arm then spirals clockwise toward the inside section of their elbow and you repeat the pressing action with stepping. Continue to practice this exercise until you are both able to execute the movements smoothly and in a continuous motion. Once you have completed this action for the right hand, place your left legs forward and repeat this exercise for the left hand.

Stepping. In the next set of exercises you practice stepping while executing the small rollback (xiao lü, 小攦) technique. Stepping allows you the opportunity to evade your opponent's attack and set yourself up in a better position to attack. In addition, it presents you with more areas to attack. Keep in mind there are many ways to go about stepping. We encourage you to explore different combinations of stepping with your partner as you become more comfortable with the movements involved. We are going to explain only one method.

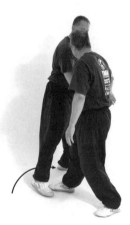

Face your partner with your right legs forward. Place the wrists so they are touching on the outside section of each other. Spiral your right hand over your partner's. Place your left leg to your left and slightly aft of your position while you perform the rollback technique.

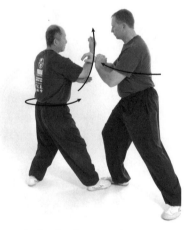

Slide your right leg back toward your left leg in preparation to step forward and attack your partner. Place the right leg forward and apply your pressing technique by sliding your left hand onto your right wrist and shifting your weight forward.

Your partner now applies wardoff (peng, 掤) and rollback (lü, 攦) to the incoming force while spiraling around your right arm and stepping to their left using their left leg followed by their right leg. Next, they slide their left hand up their right wrist and step toward you while applying press (ji, 擠). From this position you repeat the exercise back and forth until it has become smooth and continuous. Once you have done this, place the left leg forward and repeat the exercise using the opposite hand for rollback and press.

Tips to Avoid Common Errors. The most common errors for this exercise begin with not applying wardoff (peng, 掤) while neutralizing the incoming force. At this stage of training your body should be very familiar with the feeling of the wardoff (peng, 掤) structure. Another issue is incorrect stepping. Stepping allows you to further neutralize the incoming attack and positions you at a better angle to counterattack. Although we are focused on stepping to the left and slightly aft in this exercise, you may find other opportunities for stepping. Just be aware of not exposing yourself to further attack. You also need to be aware of keeping your elbow down when applying the press technique. A common error is to apply this technique with the elbow up and away from the body. This causes a loss of structure and is not as effective when applying press. Additionally, you need to be sure to keep your elbow down with the palm facing toward you when you spiral over your opponent's forearm ending at the elbow. This action is a yang circling movement.

2. Mixed (Hun He, 混合)

The next exercise involves applying the rollback technique followed by press technique to either side of your opponent. You may practice this while standing in the ma bu position first to get used to neutralizing to either side then change to the rocking positions. Finally, you practice this while stepping. Here we will describe the rocking position.

To practice this exercise, face your partner with the right legs forward. Place your right wrist on the outside section of your partner's wrist and begin to perform the rollback action. As you begin to apply your press action to your partner, they will turn the body to the right to perform the roll back movement on that side. Their left hand intercepts and spirals counterclockwise around your right arm up to your elbow. Then they slide their right hand to their left wrist to apply press toward you. You then apply your small rollback (xiao lü, 小攦) technique to either the left or right side and return with press from that side.

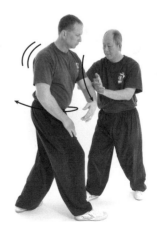

For each of these neutralizations, you will step to the left with the left leg, or to the right with the right leg, then step forward with the opposite leg to apply the press technique. You and your partner should practice this exercise until you both are able to perform the small rollback (xiao lü, 小挒) technique to either side in a continuous motion.

5.3 Large Rollback and Press

1. Rollback (Lü, 挒)

In this next section, we will describe the actions involved in the exercise of large rollback (da lü, 大挒) training. Large rollback training also contains various options of neutralizing and attacking.

In order to keep in line with the DVD series, we will describe the first set of training exercises without the press technique. Afterward we will describe the movement with the option of pressing. Although the pressing technique after rollback is not demonstrated in the DVD series, it is equally important to train. The first set of exercises will utilize the number-1 elbow neutralization explained earlier in this section.

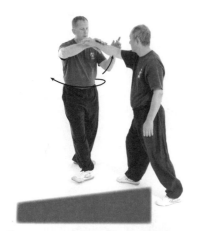 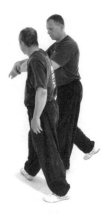

Face your partner. Pluck your partner's right wrist with your right hand while stepping toward their empty door. This may be either in front or behind your partner. You will find that directing the rollback toward the backside of your partner will require more stepping and then executing the rollback to your partner's front side.

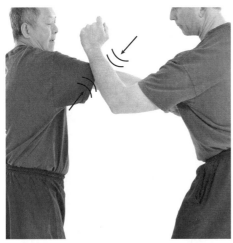
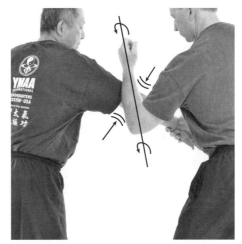

As you begin to pluck your partner's right arm, place your left forearm just above their elbow. Place the radius and ulna of your forearm so they are parallel to your partner's tendon then rotate the forearm as you apply pressure into the tendon. This attack point is known as the tianjing (TB-10) (天井) cavity and is the focal point of this particular attack.

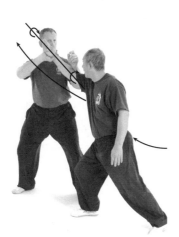

Continue to pluck your partner's arm while grinding the tendon. Your partner neutralizes the attack and returns with large rollback (da lü, 大捋). To perform this task, your partner first neutralizes the attack on the right arm by rotating the forearm and lowering their right elbow. This is immediately followed with a wardoff (peng, 掤) action toward the attacker with the right arm.

Next, they step accordingly toward your empty door, either to your front or back, and execute the same large rollback (da lü, 大捋) technique to your right arm. You then neutralize the attack on the right arm followed by applying large rollback (da lü, 大捋) to your partner's right arm once again. Continue to practice this exercise back and forth until it has become a continuous fluid motion with proper execution of the neutralization techniques. Be sure to execute the rollback for both the front side of your partner as well as the backside.

The next set of exercises for large rollback (da lü, 大捋) demonstrates the second elbow neutralization explained earlier in this section. As we have explained, this particular attack differs in the way the person initially reacts to a rollback. Their neutralization also changes slightly due to the elbow being in a bent position rather than straight.

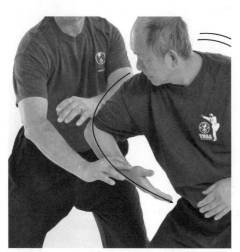

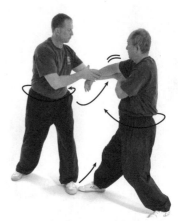

Face your partner. Your right leg is forward, and your partner's left leg is forward. Begin the large rollback (da lü, 大 攦) exercise. This time your partner bends their arm at the elbow, making it less possible to perform a lock on the elbow where you grind the cavity. Your attack point focuses on locking the inside section of your partner's arm just above the elbow. The cavity in this region is known as the shaohai (H-3, 少海) cavity. The movement is known as small elbow wrap and attacks the elbow on a different angle.

Step either toward the front or rear side of your partner's empty door while simultaneously sliding your left forearm up under your partner's right elbow. You then move your right hand back toward your body while maintaining the plucking action on their right wrist. Your left arm moves slightly forward of your partner's vertical seam and you twist your body clockwise in order to take your partner down.

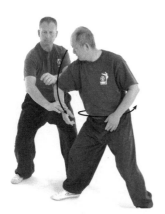

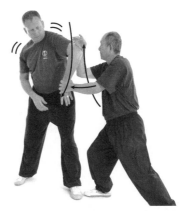

As this rollback action is being applied to your partner, they neutralize the attack using the following methods. Your partner twists their body while forming the wardoff technique and simultaneously moving their right arm toward their left hip.

Next, your partner turns back toward you while moving their right hand toward your left elbow. Their left hand moves up and begins to pluck your left hand as they simultaneously step toward your empty door, either front or back.

Finally, they slide their right forearm up just above your left elbow and apply the large rollback (da lü, 大擺) technique to you. It is now up to you to neutralize the attack as your partner has and repeat your large rollback (da lü, 大擺) to your partner's right arm. As you can see, we are only attacking the same side in these exercises. Practice this exercise using the opposite arms as well. In the next section we incorporate the use of exchanging hands and attacking the opposite sides. For now, continue to practice this action until you are both able to perform the technique smoothly for both the front and back sides of the empty door.

Tips to Avoid Common Errors. When practicing the large rollback (da lü, 大擺) technique be aware of stepping properly to achieve the correct angle for attacking the empty door. If you are not in your partner's empty door, the rollback goes into the partner's rooted foot. This mistake is more common as the attacks speed up. Another common mistake is to focus too much on the plucking action of the rollback rather than the grinding of the elbow. This pulling action requires more of a muscular effort and your partner's elbow will not be properly locked. When applied correctly, you use less muscular effort and the take down is more effortless. Finally, you must be sure to neutralize your elbow and apply wardoff (peng, 掤) energy properly to your opponent before you step toward them for the counterattack. Without applying wardoff (peng, 掤) prior to the step, your opponent is able to bump you.

2. Press (Ji, 擠)

There is one last addition to this exercise not presented on the DVD series and it adds the movement of press. There is more than one place you may apply press. You may even elect to practice this exercise without the rollback section. For this particular exercise there are two areas you can press. One area occurs immediately after you apply rollback and the other occurs immediately following your neutralization of the rollback being applied to you. We will describe these two areas here in this section.

The first method of applying press to your rollback training is to use it immediately following the application of rollback.

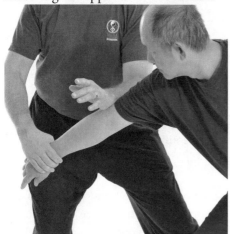 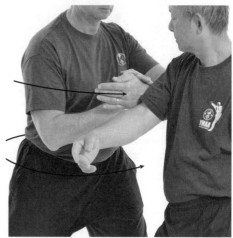

Face your partner and begin the large rollback (da lü, 大攦) training exercise. When it is your turn to apply large rollback (da lü, 大攦) immediately slide your plucking hand up toward the wrist of your opposite hand and apply press.

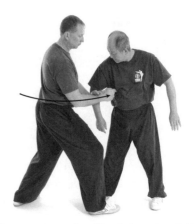

When using small rollback (xiao lü, 小攦) you can attack cavities.

You and your partner should practice applying the press technique back and forth until you both can execute the movements as a continuous flow following the rollback.

The second method is how to use the press technique immediately following your neutralization technique when rollback has been applied to you.

To begin the exercise of large rollback (da lü, 大攦), face your partner and begin the large rollback (da lü, 大攦) training exercise.

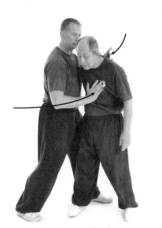

Press can also be applied as squeeze.

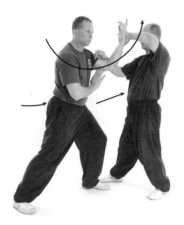

As your partner applies rollback to your arm, you neutralize the attack by rotating your forearm and dropping your elbow while applying wardoff (peng, 掤). Your arm will turn up into your partner. (You may step further into the central door if you have not already done so on the initial movement.)

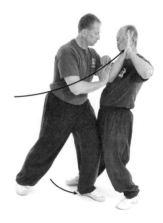

Next, place the hand of the opposite arm up onto the forearm of the neutralizing arm while placing your rear foot next to the other foot.

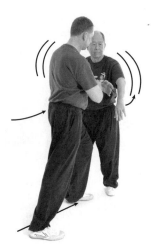

Apply press into your partner's empty door as you step through your partner's empty door.

They neutralize your press by twisting the body, applying wardoff (peng, 掤), and stepping to yield and neutralize your attack. They then return with another rollback action at which time you will once again practice the same pressing technique.

Tips to Avoid Common Errors. The most common error is improper stepping. Make sure to step into the central and empty door to place your opponent in an urgent position. You also need to pay attention to keeping your body and arm in a wardoff (peng, 掤) position as you slide the opposite hand up for attack. Additionally, the pressing action needs to be rooted while you apply it.

5.4 Mixed Rollback and Press Training

1. Changing Sides (Huan Bian, 換邊)

In this exercise you practice different combinations of the small and large rollback exercises previously described in this section. You will change between the two neutralization techniques and learn to how to apply the counterattack to both sides of each other's arms. You will also add combinations of press technique and continue to work on the various stepping techniques toward each other's front and back empty door. Continue to practice this exercise with your partner until you are both able to effortlessly use the different combinations of large or small rollback with press while stepping toward the empty doors.

Tips to Avoid Common Errors. One of the first most common errors is allowing the body to rise and sink while practicing the exercise with your partner. The body needs to be rooted as your partner applies the technique and remain rooted as you neutralize the attack. Regardless of which option of neutralization you choose to execute, be sure to apply wardoff (peng, 掤) and catch your partner's wrist with your hand to protect your sky window from being attacked. Additionally, be sure to execute the rolling of the forearm on your partner's tendon above the elbow. Do not rush the exercise. As students speed up the exercise, there is an incorrect tendency to pull the arm. To avoid this tendency, focus on the rollback action. Finally, pay careful attention to your stepping. Be sure to step so that you occupy your partner's empty door, either on the front side or the back side.

5.5 Cai/Lie/Zhou/Kao International Routine

The following routine is also known as large rollback (da lü, 大擺). It is a standardized form that has been made popular in mainland China.

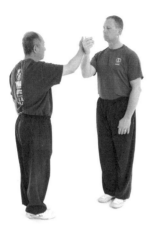

Stand facing your partner with your right hands touching at the wrist.

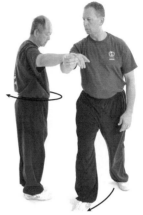

Step forward and to the left with your right foot. Your partner turns slightly as you are stepping in and this exposes them to an elbow or shoulder stroke. You begin to apply an elbow stroke toward your partner's ribcage or qimen (Li-14, 期門) cavity.

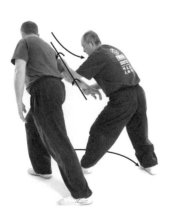

Your partner steps back into your empty door and applies large rollback (da lü, 大擺) to your attacking arm. Rollback is applied with the grinding technique applied to the tianjing (TB-10) (天井) cavity on the tendon of your elbow.

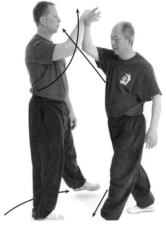

Once you feel your elbow being locked, rotate the forearm and lower the elbow for neutralizing the rollback. Your partner then begins to step forward while attacking your sky window with the right hand.

From this position you step back while twisting your body slightly to the right. Your partner begins to attack your ribcage with an elbow stroke and you then step back and apply large rollback (da lü, 大攦). Your partner now neutralizes your rollback and you begin to step forward and attack the sky window. Reaching this point, the exercise repeats itself back and forth continuously. You and your partner should continue to practice the exercise until you are both able to apply each movement correctly and fluidly.

Tips to Avoid Common Errors. Be sure to execute each movement clearly. When attacking, initially focus on the target. For training purposes this attack is similar to the movement known in the taijiquan form as strike tiger (da hu shi, 打虎勢). The second attack is an elbow stroke to the rib section. When applying the large rollback (da lü, 大攦) be sure to apply the grinding technique to the tendon of the elbow. When neutralizing the attack on the elbow, make certain that you rotate the forearm and lower the elbow. Do not lean forward when neutralizing the elbow. Finally, be careful not to rise up, moving back and forth. You should remain relatively level in height to stay rooted throughout the exercise.

5.6 Freestyle Moving Pushing Hands

The routines and theories provided so far are the basic techniques and concepts needed to deal with various situations in combat. Practicing these routines will help you build your body memory and reflexes; however, they do not provide you a deeper aspect of stepping and strategy, and they do not offer you the important training for a high level of alertness, awareness, and corresponding reaction. These routine practices are just like dancing with a partner. You are cooperating with each other and there is no real sense of enemy. In a real situation, your opponent will treat you as an enemy and will attempt to actually harm you.

In order to build up a capability for taijiquan combat, you need to practice freestyle moving pushing hands. Freestyle moving pushing hands is the door to enter actual taijiquan combat. It provides you not just techniques practice, but also stepping, angling, and learning how to set up good strategies. Most important of all, it helps you build a high level of awareness and alertness. Awareness and alertness are two crucial keys of winning in any competition.

In freestyle moving pushing hands, you improve on your basic skills such as keeping a proper distance and knowing how to adhere, listen, follow, and neutralize. You also develop your skill at setting up advantageous strategies, opening the windows, and stepping into the empty doors. Once you have all of these requirements, you should learn to apply wrestling into the pushing hands and try to take your opponent down or make them lose balance. Whenever your opponent loses their balance, root, and stability, their mind will be on regaining balance. This will allow you to create an advantageous opportunity for other attacks such as kicking and punching.

After you have mastered the skills involved in applying wrestling in moving pushing hands, you should then add qin na (擒拿) and learn how to use it to immobilize your opponent. It is very common that qin na and wrestling are used hand in hand. At this stage, you may add kicking and striking into moving pushing hands. When you have reached this stage, you are in taijiquan free sparring.

However, you should know that there is still one drill missing to lead from pushing hands to sparring. That is intercepting or attaching (zhan, 沾) in taijiquan sparring. As mentioned earlier, attaching is the skill of intercepting your opponent's incoming attacks and immediately adhering to his arms or body. This training is very important since your opponent will not be in the pushing hands situation to begin with. Most likely sparring initiates from a punch or a kick. If you're not skilled at intercepting the coming attack and setting up the pushing hands situation, you will not have any chance to use your high skills of pushing hands techniques.

This chapter only offers you an idea of how taijiquan training proceeds to the final stage of fighting capability. Due to this book's limited scope, we do not intend to get deeper in taijiquan sparring. However, in next chapter, we will offer you some concepts of how martial applications can be applied to taiji pushing hands.

Procedures from Pushing Hands to Sparring

Single Pushing Hand → Double Moving Pushing Hands → Add Rollback and Press → Apply Controlling and Borrow Jings → Add Wrestling → Add Qin Na → Add Striking and Kicking

Chapter 6: Examples of Martial Applications in Taiji Pushing Hands

6.1 Introduction

Taijiquan martial techniques contain four categories of fighting techniques: kicking, striking, wrestling, and qin na (ti, da, shuai, na; 踢、打、摔、拿). That means almost all movements were created with the possibility of applying these four categories in a battle. Therefore, as a martial taijiquan practitioner, you should understand and familiarize yourself with these four categories of skills. Even after you understand the theory and techniques, it does not mean you are able to fight. You must know how to apply it while engaging your opponent. You still need partners to train with so you are able to build your reflexes. Remember, when you are in battle, you will not have time to think. You must react without thinking. Once you have developed your reflexes and are able to react accurately and automatically, you need to accumulate experience. Since there are so many possible applications, it is impossible to introduce all of them in this book. However, we will demonstrate some typical examples for your reference. From these references you will get an idea of how to search for other techniques by yourself.

We have previously mentioned that taiji pushing hands provides the bridge to applying the knowledge of the sequence in action for freestyle fighting. Over time, you will expand your knowledge of taijiquan through the practice of a taijiquan fighting set. This eighty-eight-form structured fighting set allows the individual to apply the techniques of pushing hands training and further deepen knowledge of taiji fighting. If you wish to explore the taiji fighting set, please refer to the book *Tai Chi Martial Applications* and the DVD, *Tai Chi Fight Set* by YMAA Publication Center.

Before we describe the training exercises, we will introduce a few theories about the Thirteen Postures written by various taijiquan masters. One cannot deny the importance of knowing the Thirteen Postures and the applications of such. At this level of training, you should already have some fundamental knowledge of these Thirteen Postures and how to apply them for martial techniques. If not, it is highly recommended you refer to other books on this material as we will not go into a detailed description of them here. You can find this subject explored in detail in many of the taijiquan books available at YMAA Publication Center. In addition to the theories of the Thirteen Postures, we would like to introduce you to a few theories and the common terminology used in taijiquan fighting such as the concepts of empty doors and windows as well as rings and circles. These are common terms of which the taijiquan practitioner should be aware when training with a partner in pushing hands as well as when applying strategies in taijiquan martial application.

> The Thirteen Postures, (are derived) according to the theory of five elements and eight trigrams. They are the thirteen total jings of pushing hands. There are not another Thirteen Postures. The five elements are advance, retreat backward, beware of the left, look to the right, and central equilibrium. They can be interpreted by dividing into internal and external. Those applied to external are advance forward, retreat backward, beware of the left, look to the right, and central equilibrium. Those applied to the internal are attaching, connecting, adhering, following, and not lose contact and not resist.[1]
>
> 十三勢者，按五行八卦原理，即推手之十三種總勁，非另有十三個姿勢。五行者，即進、退、顧、盼、定之謂。分為內外兩解。行於外者，即前進、後退、左顧、右盼、中定。行於內者，即粘、連、黏、隨、不丟頂。

In this passage Master Wu, Gong-Zao (吳公藻) speaks of the Thirteen Postures being related to taiji pushing hands. Taijiquan was developed from the theory of yin and yang. We know that yin and yang are two opposite poles which, as described by Master Wong, Zong-Yue (王宗岳), divides when in motion. Yin and yang divide into four phases and, in turn, the four phases divide into eight trigrams. These eight trigrams correspond to the eight basic moving patterns of taijiquan. Just as eight postures of the thirteen are related to eight trigrams, five of the postures are related to five elements. These elements are metal (jin, 金), wood (mu, 木), water (shui, 水), fire (huo, 火), and earth (tu, 土). Each element corresponds to the Five Steppings of taijiquan. Master Wu continues to describe the internal aspects and external aspects of the Five Steppings. The pushing hands practitioner and taijiquan martial artist must be able to combine the internal and external aspects of the five postures (steppings) smoothly in order to gain the advantage over the opponent.

> The secret of thirteen total postures, few people have learned since ancient times. (Those) who have the predestined relationship (with me) have a deep fortune (today), (I) break the rules and tell you (this secret). Arc the arms, must be round and alive (i.e., peng jing), (when) the hands go out (i.e., contact with the

opponent), (first) ask the feeling (i.e., ting jing). When opponent ('s power) is void I press (i.e., ji jing) and when the opponent ('s power) is solid, (I) sink (my) elbow and repel (i.e., hua jing). Wardoff diagonally (i.e., lie jing) upward from outside, (the opponent) will lean backward and cannot stand firmly.[2]

十三總勢訣，自古少人學。

有緣深造化，破格為君說。

掤臂要圓活，出手問知覺。

敵空使我擠，敵實墜肘撥。

由外斜掤上，後仰站不著。

Master Li, Yi-She (李亦畬) tells us that few individuals have learned the true essence of taijiquan postures. He goes on to say that he will break the rules of secrecy and expose strategies of the Thirteen Postures. For instance, he explains the nature of wardoff energy (peng jing, 掤勁) with respect to arcing the arms in a round manner and keeping the movement alive, not just remaining in a stagnate position. Once again, we see the reference to making contact and listening to the opponent's power or intent. When they are void of power you may apply press jing (ji jing, 擠勁), and if they are solid you may drop your elbow and neutralize this force with redirection. Finally, you will see the reference to warding off diagonally from the outside to uproot your opponent (i.e., diagonal flying; xie fei shi, 斜飛勢).

When encountering the opponent's peng (i.e., wardoff) do not enter the territory (i.e., formed in his arcing arms). (When this happens), to attach and adhere (with the opponent) without separating is really difficult. To shut off the peng you must use the cai (i.e., pluck) and lie (i.e., split). When these two techniques have become real (i.e., succeeded), (the opponent will be) urgent without rescue. An (i.e., push) can be used to firm the four sides; consequently, the corners have different variations. Once attaching with (opponent's) hands, immediately occupy the most (advantageous position) first. Lü (i.e., rollback) and ji (i.e., press) two techniques should be applied when the opportunities allow. When zhou (i.e., elbow) and kao (i.e., bump) are used to attack, the heels are ahead first (i.e., techniques follow stepping). When there is an opportunity and an advantageous position, advance forward and retreat backward (to seize the opportunity). Gu (i.e., beware to the left) and pan (i.e., look to the right) are used within one third front and two thirds rear of attention. The solid power of the entire body depends on the yi (i.e., mind) and ding (i.e., central equilibrium). (The skills of) ting (i.e., listening jing) and probe (the opponent's intention) (i.e., understanding jing), follow, and (then) neutralize are all related to the spirit and qi. (When) seeing the (opponent's) firmness, (I) do not attack (but) gain (i.e., keep) my offensive situation (i.e., advantageous position). The day that the gongfu can be accomplished is (the day) when the entire body acts as a complete unit. (If) training without following the applications of the body (i.e., postures), (even) have cultivated (i.e., trained) until the end (i.e., death) the art is (still) hard to refine.[3]

逢手遇掤莫入盤，粘沾不離得著難。

閉掤要上採挒法，二把得實急無援。

按定四正隅方變，觸手即占先上先。

攦擠二法趁機使，肘靠攻在腳跟前。

遇機得勢進退走，三前七星顧盼間。

周身實力意中定，聽探順化神氣關。

見實不上得攻手，何日功夫是體全。

操練不按體中用，修到終期藝難精。

Master Yang, Yu (Ban-Hou) (楊鈺) (班侯) explains the application of the Thirteen Postures of taijiquan. Strategies are given such as the use of wardoff (peng jing, 掤勁) and the difficult nature of sticking with someone who applies this posture. About applying wardoff (peng jing, 掤勁), he mentions the use of pluck (cai jing, 採勁) and split (lie jing, 挒勁) to dissolve it and lead the opponent away from being centered. He continues with the use of push (an jing, 按勁) for sealing as well as the use of rollback (lü jing, 攦勁) and press (ji jing, 擠勁) being used in succession when the opportunity arises. Elbow (zhou, 肘) and bump (kao, 靠) are also mentioned along with the importance of keeping your central equilibrium while stepping to apply such forces. Finally, he places emphasis on the mind, spirit, and body training. Each is a separate component but they all act as one as the student continuously trains applications to reach a high level of skill. One should be cautious when engaging an opponent of high skill level. Knowing the opponent's skill is accomplished through listening and understanding.

6.1.1 The Three Different Fighting Ranges and Circles

It is easy to retreat from (the taiji) circle and hard to enter (the taiji) circle. When retreating or advancing, do not part (from the rules) that the waist (is loose) and (the head is) suspended upward. The most difficult is to keep the earth center (i.e., torso upright, central equilibrium) without losing its (adequate) position (i.e., posture). Retreating is easy and advancing is hard; (this saying) should be studied carefully. This is the gong (i.e., gongfu) of moving instead of stationary. Keep the body close (to the opponent's) when advancing and retreating and also compared with his shoulders (i.e., keep the same height). (You should) be able to be move like a water mill, fast or slow (as wished). The cloud dragon and the wind tigers (i.e., action of yin and yang), the appearances are round and spinning. (If you) wish to apply the heavenly circle (i.e., taiji circle), (you must) start to search now. After a long, long (time of practice), it will become natural.[4]

退圈容易進圈難，不離腰頂後與前。

所難中土不離位，退易進難仔細研。

此為動工非站定，倚身進退並比肩。

能如水磨催急緩，雲龍風虎象周旋。

要用天盤從此覓，久而久之出天然。

In this passage Yang, Yu (Ban-Hou) (楊鈺) (班侯) explains the concepts of the taiji circle and the importance of training the action of retreating and advancing. Generally speaking, Chinese martial arts contain three different fighting ranges based upon their style and strategy. These different ranges or circles are: long (長), medium (中), and short (短). Opponents who are in the long range of fighting are considered to be in the safest position because neither one of you are able to make contact without stepping or hopping forward. This distance is beyond the reach of the legs.

As you and your opponent close the distance between each other to where you both are able to reach each other by kicking, this distance is considered the medium range or circle and is more dangerous than before. In this range, one of you can cause the other to be in a defensive position by attacking first or faking an attack to create an opportunity to close into the short range or circle.

The short range or circle is when both you and your opponent are so close that either of you can reach the other simply by extending an arm. This range is considered the most dangerous. It requires you both to be extremely alert. Attacks can occur with incredible speed and travel a short distance to make contact.

Ideally, you want to remain in a long-range distance and close to the medium or short-range distance when the opportunity arises. Once you are in the medium and short ranges, you must react immediately to any change. This strategy also applies to taijiquan fighting. The difference is that taijiquan uses defense as the offense and you usually must wait for your opponent to attack before reacting. Once your opponent attacks you, use your hands to intercept and stick to the attack. Then you can shorten the distance between you and your opponent from the long range into the medium and short ranges, and at the same time you can adhere your hands to his arms or body. In taiji pushing hands training, you learn how to stick and adhere, and practice how to destroy your opponent's balance. Once your opponent loses his balance and his mind focuses on regaining it, immediately separate the adhering hands and attack. From this you can see that taijiquan fighting strategy and methods are different from most external styles in which sticking and adhering are not the main training objectives. There is an ancient document by Yang, Yu (Ban-Hou) (楊鈺) (班侯) that talks about different circles.

It is the hardest to understand the techniques of random ring. The top and the bottom follow (each other) harmoniously, its marvelousness is unlimited. Trap the enemy deeply into the random ring and (use) four ounces (to repel) a thousand pounds, the techniques are then completed. The hands and feet enter together and search for (the opportunity) in the horizontal and vertical (movements). The falling (i.e., attack) of the random ring in the palms will not be empty. If (you) wish to know what are the techniques (used) in the ring, emitting, falling, pointing (i.e., cavity press), and matching, (then) immediately successful.[5]

亂環術法最難通，上下隨合妙無窮。

陷敵深入亂環內，四兩千斤著法成。

手腳齊進橫豎找，掌中亂環落不空。

欲知環中法何在，發落點對即成功。

Here again Yang, Yu (Ban-Hou) (楊鈺) (班侯) discusses the value of what is known as the rings and the importance of producing random, variable movements to confuse your opponent in order to execute your techniques more effectively. These rings are also known in taijiquan as large (大), medium (中), and small (小) circles.

Realistically speaking, it will be hard to maintain contact or adhere to your opponent while solely using this technique. A more viable action would be to shrink your circling action to a medium circle (zhong quan, 中圈).

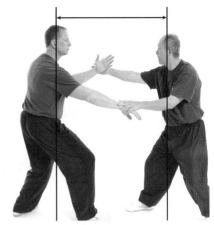

When engaging your opponent while using a long extended arm circling technique, you are performing within a large circle (da quan, 大圈).

Within the medium circle range, your arms have better ability to extend or withdraw and you are more easily able to maintain contact with your opponent. In this circle, you have to compete with your opponent to see who is more capable of destroying the other's balance, thus creating an opportunity for attack.

Finally. there is the small circle (xiao quan, 小圈).

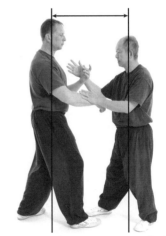

In the medium circle (zhong quan, 中圈), your arms are half bent and the adhering maneuvers become much easier and more practical.

To maneuver within the small circle, your skills must be very high and you must be very alert to your opponent's actions. These actions often occur in short range and can be so fast it is almost impossible to react to the movement. This is why it is said, "The higher the skills are, the smaller the circle will be."

6.1.2 Sky and Ground Windows (天窗、地窗)

When you are in a combat situation, you must always be aware of two important concepts: empty doors and windows. Since we have mentioned the concepts of doors previously in chapter 4 under the moving single pushing hands section, we will not repeat the description here.

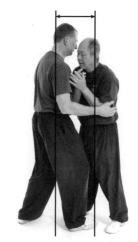

In the small circle (xiao quan, 小圈), the action can be considered coiling or spiraling.

The other concept of importance to taijiquan practitioners is the window (chuang, 窗). Windows are areas on you and your opponent that are exposed to attack. Generally speaking, there are the sky window (tian chuang, 天窗) and the ground window (di chuang, 地窗).

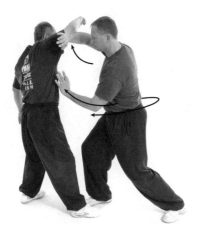

Fair Lady Weaves with Shuttle (yu nü chuan suo, 玉女穿梭) is an example of a technique that can be used to expose the ground window for attack.

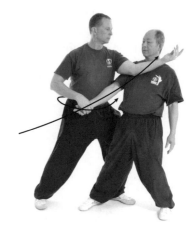

Diagonal flying (xie fei shi, 斜飛勢) is an example of a technique that can be used to expose the sky window for attack.

In order to attack through a window, you must open it and then attack immediately. Usually you can open the opponent's window easily, but he can close it just as easily. It is for this reason that you must have a good foundation of the concepts of substantial and insubstantial. A very skilled opponent will attempt to apply their techniques while keeping their doors closed. You will need to expose these areas through the use of strategies of insubstantial and substantial intentions.

6.2 Kicking in Taiji Pushing Hands

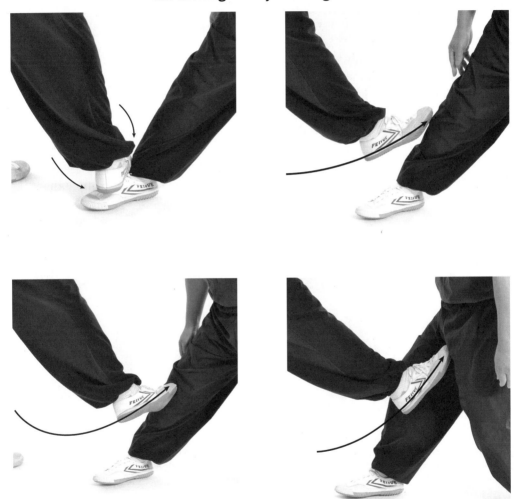

Examples of kicking.

The first of the four fighting categories we will review is kicking (ti, 踢). Kicking can be either the technique of using the foot to attack your opponent's critical areas or using your foot to trip them. A skillful fighter will understand how to mutually exchange punching and kicking techniques. Taijiquan is a style that focuses on the middle- and short-range fighting techniques. When you attack the opponent, the focus of the kick will be on the opponent's foot, shins, knees, as well as the groin. Kicks must be quick while maintaining proper rooting. You also need to remain aware of protecting your own vital areas. Throughout the interaction, you need to be able to sense your opponent's intention to kick you. Taijiquan techniques also focus on remaining attached and listening. When this occurs, you will use techniques such as pressing, pulling, bumping, or any other wrestling technique necessary to destroy their balance and root.

We will demonstrate only a few techniques to further illustrate the methods of kicking in pushing hands. As mentioned, there are many techniques of kicking, punching, wrestling, and qin na hidden within the movements of taijiquan and pushing hands. Continue to train and explore other opportunities on your own.

The first technique of kicking is demonstrated off the double push hands neutralization. Stand facing your partner, right leg forward, and begin your double push hands neutralization back and forth. All neutralizations should be practiced. Next, you should practice your neutralization with a kick. Choose your neutralization and apply the kick.

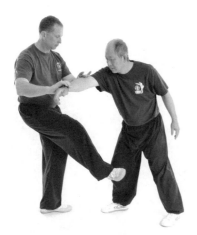

While using the horizontal neutralization, you may use your right leg from the aft position to kick your opponent.

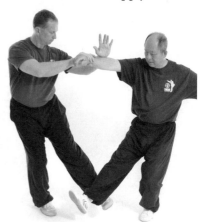

While using your horizontal neutralization you may also use your left foot from the forward position to kick your opponent's leg.

Practice, exchanging kicks with your partner. The entry into a kick should be smooth and your intention should not be obvious to your partner. With continued practice, you should begin to be able to sense your partner's actions and be able to counter their kicking techniques.

Also train using large rollback (da lü, 大攦) or wardoff (peng, 掤), rollback (lü, 攦), press (ji, 擠), and push (an, 按) techniques to practice kicking.

6.3 Striking in Taiji Pushing Hands

Striking is defined as using the hand to punch, cut, slide, hammer, or point. There are many hand strikes with various hand forms. Other than kicking, striking (da, 打) is the most common technique that a martial artist must master. This is because some basic level of striking techniques is easier to train and can be fast and effective. From past martial art fighting experience, it is known that as long as you have speed and strong power in executing your striking techniques, you have already won half the battle. However, how you manifest the speed and power to its higher efficiency remains the crucial key of winning.

As mentioned in previous chapters, there are many forms of jing manifestation. Taijiquan is a middle- to short-range style of fighting that emphasizes soft jing and targeting in cavity strikes (dian xue, 點穴). Effective cavity strikes also require knowing where and when to strike the cavities. However, you should also understand a proficient martial artist cannot just execute soft jing skillfully but must also have the skill of applying soft-hard and hard jing as well.

In order to execute the strike, one must understand how to apply yin-yang coiling jing and controlling jing in order to create the proper situation for striking the sky window (tian chuang, 天窗) or the ground wicket (di hu, 地戶) (di chuang, 地窗). Of course, you also need to be able to step correctly to enter the central door (zhong men, 中門) and attack your opponent's empty door (kong men, 空門) to create the best opportunity for attack. Through pushing hands training, you learn how to create an advantageous position for this type of attacking. Keep in mind that you also need to be aware of your vulnerability to attack. Even though you create an opportunity for attack, your opponent, if skilled, will also apply their coiling and controlling techniques while remaining attached to you.

In the following section, we will demonstrate a few techniques for striking while performing taiji pushing hands. Once again, there are too many techniques to cover them all.

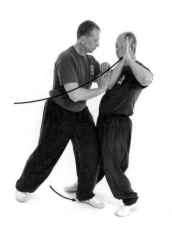

Neutralize with small rollback (xiao lü, 小 擴) while stepping into your opponent's empty door. Step into their open door and use press (ji, 擠) for striking the solar plexus

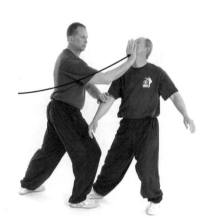

Use a downward neutralization. Your left hand coils over your opponent's right wrist, moving to seal your opponent's elbow. Your right hand will now be able to strike your opponent's sky window.

Face your partner with the right leg forward and begin to practice the double push hands neutralization while stationary. Continue to practice all the techniques of double hands neutralization for a warm up. Next, perform the downward neutralization. Allow the left hand to coil over the opponent's elbow while simultaneously performing a yang coil over your partner's right wrist. Your left hand will seal your partner's elbow down and the right hand will now be able to strike your partner's sky window.

The next exercise will be done while performing large rollback (da lü, 大擴). Step into position with your partner and begin practicing moving large rollback (da lü, 大擴). Allow your partner to begin their attack and neutralize it with small rollback (xiao lü, 小擴) while stepping into their empty door. This will allow you to step into their open door and use press (ji, 擠) for striking the solar plexus.

6.4 Wrestling in Taiji Pushing Hands

The next technique is wrestling. It is considered as important as kicking and punching, and in the right situation it can play an important role in winning. This was especially true in ancient battle periods where almost all warriors wore armor and helmets. Under this situation, it would not be easy for anyone to kill their opponent with weapons or bare hands. However, if the opponent was on the ground, areas such as neck, armpits, waist, and groin, which were normally protected by draper net, would be exposed. Once the opponent was on the ground it would take them time to get up again due to the weight of the helmet and armor. Their defense capability would be greatly weakened. When this happened, it would allow time to kill your opponent. The final goal of the ancient warrior was to eliminate the enemy as soon as possible and eliminate as many of them as possible.

Wrestling is a defensive technique generally used when an opponent strikes or kicks you. Taijiquan focuses on middle to short-range fighting. Your opponent is also looking for the opportunity to enter the central door and attack. Using the skills of listening, attaching, adhering, and following, you look to destroy your opponent's root and take the opponent down. Keep in mind that you must have good balance and rooting in order to apply the wrestling techniques. Otherwise your opponent will be able to apply wrestling techniques on you. If you find yourself in this situation it is necessary to sink your center of gravity downward to firm your root through turning and rotating. You also need to use wardoff jing to protect your center.

The following exercises are performed while using the moving double pushing hands neutralization. In order to practice the techniques, you need to have knowledge of wrestling techniques. It is recommended you review the wrestling techniques on the DVD, *Taiji Wrestling—Advanced Takedown Techniques*, by Dr. Yang, Jwing-Ming and available from YMAA Publication Center.

Face your partner and begin practicing the stationary double push hands exercise. When comfortable, you will neutralize your partner's incoming force. While neutralizing the incoming force, you need to step into the central door as well as the empty door and apply your wrestling technique. The following are a few examples of takedowns that can be utilized after neutralizing an attack.

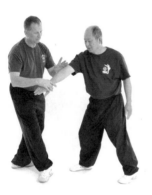 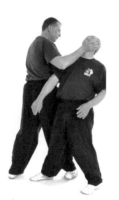 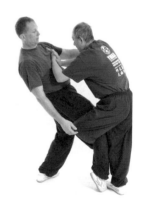

A few examples of takedowns that can be utilized after neutralizing an attack.

6.5 Controlling in Taiji Pushing Hands

Qin na (擒拿) is an effective technique against an opponent's grab and is used for short-range fighting situations. As mentioned in the last section, wrestling is the technique that can take your opponent to the ground. However, in order to execute a wrestling technique, you often need to grab your opponent's body to effectively apply the wrestling technique. Qin na was developed against this grabbing. Since taijiquan is considered a middle to short-range fighting style, it also makes use of qin na techniques. In this section, we will first summarize qin na theory in a thesis. After that, a few examples of qin na techniques will be shown to give you an idea of how qin na can be used in taijiquan fighting.

Qin na consists of five categories. They are dividing the muscle/tendons, misplacing the bones, sealing the breath, sealing the arteries, and cavity strikes. Most beginners will only learn misplacing the bone and dividing the muscle/tendons before gaining the proper skills to advance to cavity strikes. Initially their movements will be generated more from a muscular force and easily detected and countered. Over time, the body will learn how to move more correctly, breathing will become more natural, and qi will flow more freely. Since the application of qin is so smooth and natural for qin na experts, it is usually not easy for their opponents to forecast their techniques.

Qin na techniques are applied differently in taijiquan than in external styles. They are more rounded and utilize the soft techniques of neutralizing and controlling angles. It is important to practice the listening, following, adhering, and attaching jings skills in order to effectively apply qin na techniques.

The following figures are examples of different options you have while practicing the horizontal neutralization of the double push hands exercises.

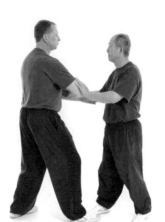 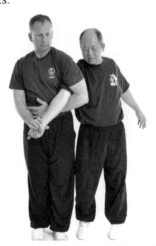

Examples of different qin na options after using the horizontal neutralization of the double push hands exercises.

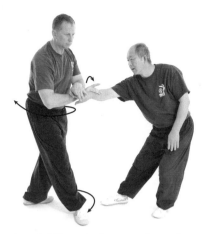 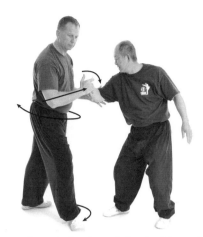

Examples of different qin na options after using the horizontal neutralization of the double push hands exercises.

In order to practice the qin na techniques while practicing pushing hands, it is recommended that you have knowledge of qin na techniques. These techniques can be reviewed on the book and DVD, *Taiji Chin Na in Depth—The Seizing Art of Taijiquan,* by Dr. Yang, Jwing-Ming available from YMAA Publication Center. Due to the endless options of qin na techniques that may be applied while using the push hands exercises, we will not describe the actions in detail in this book. You will need to practice your push hands exercises with a partner and explore the various qin na applications available while neutralizing the incoming forces.

References

1. Dr. Yang, Jwing-Ming, *Tai Chi Secrets of the Wu Style* (太極拳吳氏先哲祕要) (Wolfeboro, NH: YMAA Publication Center, 2002), 6.

2. Dr. Yang, Jwing-Ming, *Tai Chi Secrets of the Wǔ and Li Style* (太極拳武、李氏先哲祕要) (Wolfeboro, NH: YMAA Publication Center, 2001), 75.

3. Dr. Yang, Jwing-Ming, *Tai Chi Secrets of the Yang Style* (太極拳楊氏先哲祕要) (Wolfeboro, NH: YMAA Publication Center, 2001), 17.

4. Dr. Yang, Jwing-Ming, *Tai Chi Secrets of the Yang Style* (太極拳楊氏先哲祕要), 53.

5. Dr. Yang, Jwing-Ming, *Tai Chi Secrets of the Yang Style* (太極拳楊氏先哲祕要), 24.

Chapter 7: Conclusion

Taijiquan, or the grand ultimate fist, is a martial art practiced by many in today's society. Over the years, many people have discovered the health benefits of this art. Studies have shown that taijiquan practice improves balance; benefits cognitive function; improves cardiovascular health, including blood pressure and heart rate; helps practitioners manage pain; and eases symptoms of arthritis, among other health issues. Although these undeniable benefits have helped taijiquan to become a popular form of exercise for health, it has allowed the martial value of the art to fade. Every movement of taijiquan has its unique martial purpose. Without this martial root, taijiquan practice would be just like a form of dancing, without deep meaning and feeling. Taijiquan follows the laws of yin-yang theory, and without the knowledge of martial applications this art will remain out of balance and shallow.

In an attempt to restore this balance, the authors have written this book, and several others, as tools for those who wish to ponder the depths of this art. The exercises are just one stage in learning how to train the mind and body to increase the sensitivity to your surroundings. The book is intended for use as a complement to the YMAA series of DVDs on pushing hands, taiji wrestling, and taiji qin na. Utilizing these aids, along with continued training with various partners as well as participation in seminars, provides a path to rectify mistakes, explore your questions, and attain the higher levels of taijiquan pushing hands. We encourage you to participate in seminars. Participating in seminars allows you to feel and experience the real action with partners under the guidance of qualified teachers. It is an important part of reaching new depths of understanding and skill.

Throughout this training, remember to remain humble and continue to seek further knowledge through training and research. These exercises are not an end but the beginning of your journey. The information we provide is not the sole authority of taijiquan and it is up to you how far you wish to train the mind and body.

Acknowledgements

The authors would like to thank the following: Tim Comrie for typesetting and photos, Leslie Takao and Doran Hunter for editing, Axie Breen for photos and cover design, Quentin Lopes for drawing lines in photos, Pat Rice and Nick Gracenin for their Forewords.

Appendix: Translation and Glossary of Chinese Terms

àn (按). Settle the wrist.

bá gēn (拔根). Pull the root upward.

bā mén (八門) Eight Doors. The eight basic jìng patterns of tàijíquán that handle eight corners of defense and offense.

bā mén wǔ bù (八門五步). Eight Doors and Five Steppings. Eight Doors mean the eight jìngs that are used for defense and offense. Five Steppings means five basic stepping movements in fighting.

bái hè (白鶴). White Crane. A southern style of Chinese martial arts.

bǎihuì (Gv-20) (百會). Hundred meetings. An acupuncture cavity located on the crown. It belongs to the governing vessel.

biàn jiǎo dù (變角度). Biàn means change. Jiǎo dù means angle. Change angle.

cǎi (採). Pluck. One of eight jìng patterns in the tàijíquán Thirteen Postures.

cǎi jìng (採勁). Pluck jìng. The power manifestation of cǎi.

cè huà (側化). Sideways neutralization.

chán jìng (纏勁). Coiling jìng.

chán shǒu liàn xí (纏手練習). Chán shǒu means coiling and sticking hands. Liàn xí means training or practice.

chán sī jìng (纏絲勁). Silk reeling jing (Chén style). Similar to Yáng style's yīn-yáng symbol sticking hands.

cháng (長). Long.

chōng mài (衝脈). The thrusting vessel. One of the eight qì vessel in the body.

chuāng (窗). Window.

chuí zhí (垂直). Vertical.

dà (大). Large or big.

dǎ (打). Strike.

dǎ hǔ shì (打虎勢). Strike tiger posture.

dǎ huí jìng (打回勁). Striking returning jìng. The jìng is manifested in between the end of the opponent's attack and the retreat of the attack.

dà lǚ (大擺). Large rollback.

dǎ mèn jìng (打悶勁). Striking the oppressive jìng. The other name of borrowing jìng (jiè jìng, 借勁).

dà quān (大圈). Large circle.

dà zhōu tiān (大周天). Grand qì circulation.

dān liàn (單練). Solo training.

dān shǒu (單手). Single hand.

dān tuī shǒu (單推手). Single pushing hand.

dàzhuī (Gv-14) (大椎). Big vertebra. One of the acupuncture cavities. It belongs to governing vessel.

dēng shān bù (登山步). Mountain climbing stance. One of the basic stances of the Chinese martial arts.

dì chuāng (地窗). Ground window.

dì hù (地戶). Ground wicket.

diǎn xué (點穴). Cavity strike. Diǎn means to point and xué means cavity.

dìng bù (定步). Stationary.

dìng gēn (定根). To firm the root.

dòng bù (動步). Stepping.

duǎn (短). Short.

duì dǎ/sǎn dǎ (對打／散打). Sparring.

duó qiú (奪球). Capture the ball.

fā jìng (發勁). Emitting jìng.

fàn lì (範例). Example.

fáng shāng (防傷). Injury prevention.

fū suǐ xī (膚髓息). Skin-marrow breathing. A qìgōng grand circulation practice.

Húběi Sheng (湖北省). A province in China.

gōng jiàn bù (弓箭步). Bow and arrow stance. One of the basic stances in the Chinese martial arts. It is also called dēng shān bù (登上步).

gǒng shǒu (拱手). Arcing the arms. Also commonly used for greeting.

hā (哈). The sound of manifesting power.

hǎi dǐ (海底). Sea bottom. Implies perineum.

hēng (哼). The sound of storing power.

hǔ zhǎo (虎爪). Tiger claw. A style of Chinese martial arts.

huà (化). Neutralize.

huā quán xiù tuǐ (花拳繡腿). Flower fist and brocade leg. Implies that the martial arts performed are not powerful and cannot be used in a real fight.

huàn biān (換邊). Change directions or change side.

huái zhōng bào yuè (懷中抱月). Embracing the moon on the chest. Name of a form of qìgōng practice.

huìyīn (Co-1) (會陰). Meet yīn. Perineum. Name of an acupuncture cavity. It belongs to the conceptional vessel.

hùn hé (混合). Mix together.

huǒ (火). Fire.

huó bù (活步). Alive stepping.

jǐ (擠). Squeeze or press.

jī běn (基本). Basic or fundamental.

jī běn jìng (基本勁). Basic jìngs.

jǐ huà (擠化). Press and neutralize.

jǐ jìng (擠勁). Squeeze or press jìng.

jiǎo dù gǎn (角度感). Sense of angling.

jiè jìng (借勁). Borrowing jìng. Borrowing jìng is known as the ability to sense an opponent's attacking jìng and borrow the energy before it was manifested.

jiè shaò (介紹). Introduction.

jīn (金). Metal.

jìng (勁). Power manifestation.

jìng gōng (勁功). Gōngfū of jìng's manifestation.

jīng shén (精神). The spirit of vitality.

jiūwěi (Co-15) (鳩尾). Wild pigeon's tail. Name of an acupuncture cavity. It belongs to the conception vessel.

jù gǎn (距感). Sense of distance.

kaò (靠). Bump.

Kaō, Taó (高濤). Dr. Yang, Jwing-Ming's tàijíquán master.

kōng mén (空門). Empty door. The door that allows you to attack.

kuà (胯). Hip joint area.

lán què wěi (攔雀尾). Grasp Sparrows Tail. Name of a tàijíquán posture.

laógōng (P-8) (勞宮). Labor's palace. Name of an acupuncture cavity, located at the center of the palms and belonging to the pericardium primary qì channel (xīn bāo luò jīng, 心包絡經).

lǐ lùn (理論). Theory.

Lǐ, Yì-Shē (AD 1832–1892) (李亦畬). A famous tàijíquán master during the Qīng Dynasty (AD 1644–1911) (清朝).

lián huán jìng (連環勁). Linking jìng. Jìng is manifested continuously.

liàn xí (練習). Practice or train.

liè (挒). Split.

liè jìng (挒勁). Split jìng.

liù gōng (六弓). Six bows, meaning four limbs (four bows), spine, and chest that can be used to store power for manifestation.

liù hé bā fǎ (六合八法). A style of internal Chinese martial arts, also called water style. This style is a combination of tàijíquán, xíngyìquán, and bāguàzhǎng.

liù zhuǎn jué (六轉訣). Six turning secrets.

láogōng xí (勞宮息). Laogong breathing. A gland qì circulation qìgōng practice.

lóng xíng (龍形). Dragon shape. A style of Chinese martial arts.

lǚ (攦). Rollback.

lǚ/jí (撊 / 擠). Rollback/press.

lùn tuī shǒu (論推手). Discuss pushing hands.

luò (絡). Secondary channels that branch out from the main channels to the skin and every part of the body.

luó xuán jìng (螺旋勁). Spiraling jìng.

mǎ bù (馬步). Horse stance. One of the basic stances in the Chinese martial arts.

mìngmén (Gv-4) (命門). Life door. The name of an acupuncture cavity that belongs to the governing vessel.

mù (木). Wood.

ná (拿). This means qín ná (擒拿), which means to seize and control.

ná jìng (拿勁). Controlling jìng.

nèi hán (內含). Contents.

nèi kuà (內胯). Internal kuà. Kuà means the waist and hip joints area.

niǔ zhuǎn (扭轉). Twisting.

niǔ zhuǎn jìng (扭轉勁). Twisting jìng.

péng (掤). Wardoff.

péng jìng (掤勁). Wardoff jìng.

qián hòu dòng (前後動). Forward and backward movement. Means rocking.

qiǎng kōngmén (搶空門). Occupy empty door.

qiǎng zhōng mén (搶中門). Occupy central door.

qígōng (氣功). Qí means energy and gōng means gōngfū. Qìgōng means the study or practice of energy.

qímén (Li-14) (期門). Expectation's door. Name of an acupuncture cavity that belongs to the liver channel.

qín ná (擒拿). Seize and control.

ràng (讓). Yield.

sān cái shì (三才勢). Three power posture. A standing meditation posture of tài-jíquán qígōng.

sān pán (三盤). Three sections of the body. The entire body can be divided into three sections: from the knees down, from the knees to xīnkǎn (心坎) (jiūwěi, Co-15) (鳩尾), and from xinkan to the crown.

sàn shǒu duì liàn (散手對練). Tàijí fighting set.

shā dài (沙袋). Sand bag.

shàng huà (上化). Upward neutralization.

shàohǎi (H-3) (少海). Lesser sea. Name of an acupuncture cavity that belongs to the heart channel.

shè jiǎo (設角). Set up an angle.

shé xíng (蛇形). Snake shape. A style of Chinese martial arts.

shén (神). Spirit.

shén xí (神息). Spiritual breathing.

shí sān shì (十三势). Thirteen Postures, foundation of tàijíquán.

shuāi (摔). Wrestling.

shuāng liàn (雙練). Two-person practice together.

shuāng shǒu (雙手). Two hands.

shuāng tuī jìng (雙推勁). Double push jìng.

shuāng tuī shǒu (雙推手). Double pushing hands.

shuǐ (水). Water.

shuǐ píng (水平). Horizontal.

shuǐ píng huà (水平化). Horizontal neutralization.

sì liù bù (四六步). Four-six stance. One of the basic stances in Chinese martial arts.

sì xīn xí (四心息). Four gates breathing. A martial arts grand circulation practice.

Sòng (AD 960–1279) (宋朝). A Chinese dynasty.

sōng kuà (鬆胯). Loosen up the hip area.

sōng yāo (鬆腰). Loosen up the waist area.

suí jìng (隨勁). Following jìng.

suí qì (髓氣). Marrow qì.

tàijí jìng (太極勁). Tàijí power manifestation.

tàijí qiú qìgōng (太極球氣功). Tàijí ball qìgōng.

tàijí quān (太極圈). Tàijí yīn-yáng symbol circle.

tàijí tuī shǒu (太極推手). Tàijí pushing hands.

tàijí yīn-yáng quān (太極陰陽圈). Tàijí yīn-yáng symbol circle.

tàijíquán (太極拳). Grand ultimate fist. One of the internal Chinese martial arts.

tī (踢). Kicking.

tǐ xī (體息). Body breathing. One of qìgōng's grand circulation practices.

tiān chuāng (天窗). Sky window.

tiānjǐng (TB-10) (天井). Heaven's well. One of the acupuncture cavities. It belongs to the triple burner channel (sān jiāo, 三焦).

tiāntú (Co-22) (天突). Heaven's prominence. One of the acupuncture cavities. It belongs to the conception vessel.

tīng jìng (聽勁). Listening jìng.

tóng biān (同邊). Same side.

tǔ (土). Earth.

tuī lā (推拉). Push and pull.

wài kuà (外胯). The external hip joint area.

Wáng, Zōng-Yuè (王宗岳). A famous tàijíquán master during the Qīng Dynasty (AD 1644–1911) (清朝).

wèi qì (衛氣). Guardian qì.

wèn dá (問答). Questions and answers.

wǔ bù (五步). Five strategic steppings in tàijíquán.

wǔ xīn xí (五心息). Five gates breathing. One of the grand circulation qìgōng practices of Chinese martial arts.

wǔ xué (武學). Martial scholarship.

wǔ xué yìng yòng (武學應用). Applications of martial scholarship.

Wú, Gōng-Zǎo (AD 1902–1983) (吳公藻). A well-known tàijíquán master at the beginning of the last century.

Wǔdāng (武當). Name of a mountain located in China's Húběi Province (湖北省).

wú jí (無極). No extremity. This means no polarity, nothingness, or a tiny single point in space.

Wǔ, Chéng-Qīng (AD 1800–1884) (武澄清). A famous tàijíquán master during the Qīng Dynasty (AD 1644–1911) (清朝).

Wǔ, Yǔ-Xiāng (AD 1812–1880) (武禹襄). A famous tàijíquán master during the Qīng Dynasty (AD 1644–1911) (清朝).

wǔ xíng (五行). Five phases or five elements (i.e., metal, wood, water, fire, and earth).

xǐ suǐ jīng (洗髓經). Marrow/brain washing qìgōng.

xià huà (下化). Downward neutralization.

xià pán (下盤). Lower section of the body from hips or knees down to the feet.

xià pán gōng (下盤功). Training the lower section of the body.

xiǎo (小). Small.

xiǎo lǚ (小攦). Small rollback.

xiǎo quān (小圈). Small circle.

xié fēi shì (斜飛勢). Diagonal flying. A form of tàijíquán posture.

xīn bāo luò jīng (心包絡經). Pericardium primary qì channel.

xīnkǎn (心坎). Heart pit. A cavity for martial arts striking. It is called jiūwěi (Co-15) (鳩尾) in acupuncture.

xū bù (虛步). False stance or insubstantial stance.

xū shí (虛實). Insubstantial and substantial.

xuán jī bù (玄機步). Tricky stance. It means false stance (xū bù, 虛步).

xùn liàn (訓練). Train.

yáng quān (陽圈). Yáng symbol circle.

yáng shén (陽神). Yáng spirit. Spirit that is raised up by emotional stimulation.

Yáng, Bān-Hóu (AD 1837–1890) (楊班侯). A famous tàijíquán master during the Qīng Dynasty (AD 1644–1911) (清朝). He is also called Yáng, Yù (楊鈺).

Yáng, Chéng-Fǔ (AD 1883–1936) (楊澄甫). A famous tàijíquán master during the period at the end of the Qīng Dynasty (AD 1644–1911) (清朝) and the beginning of The Republic of China (中華民國).

Yáng, Jwìng-Mǐng (楊俊敏). One of the authors of this book.

Yáng, Yù (AD 1837–1890) (楊鈺). A famous tàijíquán master during the Qīng Dynasty (AD 1644–1911) (清朝). He is also called Yáng, Bān-Hóu (楊班侯).

yì (意). Wisdom mind or logical thinking.

yì bān cuò wù (一般錯誤). Common errors.

yì jīn jīng (易筋經). Muscle/tendon changing qìgōng.

yǐn (引). Lead.

yīn quān (陰圈). Yin symbol circle.

yīn yáng (陰陽). Two opposite positions of conditions or matters. Usually, yīn is translated as deficient and yang is translated as excess in Chinese medicine.

yīn yáng quān (陰陽圈). Yīn-yáng circle.

yīn yáng zhǎn zhuǎn (陰陽輾轉). Yīn-yáng circling.

yīn-yáng huà (陰／陽化). Yīn-yáng neutralization.

yīnjiāo (Co-7) (陰交). Yīn's junction. An acupuncture cavity that belongs to the conception vessel.

yìntáng (M-HN-3) (印堂). Seal hall. A miscellaneous cavity in Chinese acupuncture.

yǒngquán (K-1) (湧泉). Gushing spring. An acupuncture cavity that belongs to the kidney qì channel.

yǒngquán xí (湧泉息). Yǒngquán qì breathing.

yǔ bàn tóng liàn (與伴同練). Train with partners.

yù nǚ chuān suō (玉女穿梭). Fair Lady Weaves with Shuttle. A posture of tàijíquán.

zhā gèn (紮根). Build a firm root.

zhān (沾). Intercept or attach.

zhān qiú (沾球). Adhering to the ball.

zhàn zhuāng (站樁). Trained on posts. It means standing meditation qìgōng practice.

Zhāng, Sān-Fēng (AD 1247–?) (張三豐). Credited as the creator of tàijíquán during the Southern Sòng Dynasty (AD 1127–1279) (南宋).

zhēn dān tián (真丹田). Real dān tián. Located at the center of gravity (i.e., physical center).

zhōng (中). Medium.

zhōng dìng (中定). Central equilibrium. One of tàijíquán's five strategic steppings.

zhōng mén (中門). Central door. The shoulder-width space between two individuals facing each other.

zhōng quān (中圈). Medium circle.

zhóu (肘). Elbow.

zhóu mǒ huà (肘抹化). Elbow smearing neutralization.

zhóu huà (肘化). Elbow neutralization.

zhóu shùn huà (肘順化). Elbow following neutralization.

zhōu tiān mài yùn gōng (周天邁運功). Martial arts grand circulation.

zhuǎn quān (轉圈). Circling.

zhuō shàng zhǎn zhuǎn (桌上輾轉). Wrap coiling on the table.

zì wǒ liàn xí (自我練習). Self-practice.

zì yóu (自由). Free. It means freestyle in this book.

zhōng tǔ (中土). Refers to central earth, or central equilibrium.

zǒu bù (走步). Walking.

zuǒ lán què wěi (左攔雀尾). Grasp Sparrow's Tail—left. One of the tàijíquán forms.

Index

About the Authors

David Grantham

David Grantham was born on September 22, 1965, in Dorchester, Massachusetts, and raised in Weymouth, Massachusetts, from the age of three. At the age of eighteen, he attended Bridgewater State College to pursue his dream of aviation and currently is employed by United Airlines as a pilot based in New Jersey.

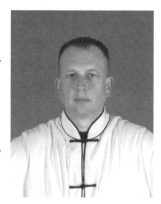

Mr. Grantham began his martial arts training at the age of twenty-four, studying hua yue tai chi (liuhebafaquan) as well as a two-person fighting form under the tutelage of instructor David Zucker. Mr. Zucker studied under the late Master John Chung Li. After training for one year with Mr. Zucker, Mr. Grantham was encouraged to further his knowledge of Chinese martial arts and it was recommended that he attend Yang's Martial Arts Association headquartered in Boston. He joined YMAA and started training the Shaolin curriculum. During his years of training at the school and attending seminars abroad, Mr. Grantham expanded his studies to include taijiquan and qigong. On January 28, 2000, he earned assistant instructor of chin na followed by the rank of chin na instructor on January 30, 2007. In 2008, Mr. Grantham earned his coach instructor position from YMAA president Nicholas Yang.

David Grantham has been training in martial arts, taijiquan, and qigong for over thirty years. He is the coauthor of the book *Tai Chi Ball Qigong* published in November of 2010. He continues to train the YMAA curriculum and currently teaches at the Hunterdon Health and Wellness Center in Clinton, New Jersey. David Grantham resides in Hunterdon County, New Jersey, with his wife, Jenifer, and two children, Jillian and Alexander.

Yang, Jwing-Ming, PhD (楊俊敏博士)

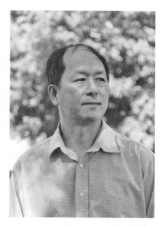

Dr. Yang, Jwing-Ming was born on August 11, 1946, in Xinzhu Xian (新竹縣), Taiwan (台灣), Republic of China (中華民國). He started his wushu (武術) (gongfu or kung fu, 功夫) training at the age of fifteen under Shaolin White Crane (Shaolin *Bai He*, 少林白鶴) Master Cheng, Gin-Gsao (曾金灶). Master Cheng originally learned taizuquan (太祖拳) from his grandfather when he was a child. When Master Cheng was fifteen years old, he started learning White Crane from Master Jin, Shao-Feng (金紹峰) and followed him for twenty-three years until Master Jin's death.

In thirteen years of study (1961–1974) under Master Cheng, Dr. Yang became an expert in the White Crane style of Chinese martial arts, which includes both the use of bare hands and various weapons, such as saber, staff, spear, trident, two short rods, and many others. With the same master he also studied White Crane qigong (氣功), qin na or chin na (擒拿), tui na (推拿), and dian xue massage (點穴按摩) and herbal treatment.

At sixteen, Dr. Yang began the study of Yang-tyle taijiquan (楊氏太極拳) under Master Kao Tao (高濤). He later continued his study of taijiquan under Master Li, Mao-Ching (李茂清). Master Li learned his taijiquan from the well-known Master Han, Ching-Tang (韓慶堂). From this further practice, Dr. Yang was able to master the taiji bare-hand sequence, pushing hands, the two-man fighting sequence, taiji sword, taiji saber, and taiji qigong.

When Dr. Yang was eighteen years old, he entered Tamkang College (淡江學院) in Taipei Xian to study physics. In college, he began the study of traditional Shaolin Long Fist (Changquan or Chang Chuan, 少林長拳) with Master Li, Mao-Ching at the Tamkang College Guoshu Club (淡江國術社), 1964–1968, and eventually became an assistant instructor under Master Li. In 1971, he completed his MS degree in physics at the National Taiwan University (台灣大學) and then served in the Chinese Air Force from 1971 to 1972. In the service, Dr. Yang taught physics at the Junior Academy of the Chinese Air Force (空軍幼校) while also teaching wushu. After being honorably discharged in 1972, he returned to Tamkang College to teach physics and resumed study under Master Li, Mao-Ching. From Master Li, Dr. Yang learned Northern Style Wushu, which includes both bare hand and kicking techniques, and numerous weapons.

In 1974, Dr. Yang came to the United States to study mechanical engineering at Purdue University. At the request of a few students, Dr. Yang began to teach gongfu, which resulted in the establishment of the Purdue University Chinese Kung Fu Research Club in the spring of 1975. While at Purdue, Dr. Yang also taught college-credit courses in taijiquan. In May of 1978, he was awarded a PhD in mechanical engineering by Purdue.

In 1980, Dr. Yang moved to Houston to work for Texas Instruments. While in Houston, he founded Yang's Shaolin Kung Fu Academy, which was eventually taken over by his disciple, Mr. Jeffery Bolt, after Dr. Yang moved to Boston in 1982. Dr. Yang founded Yang's Martial Arts Academy in Boston on October 1, 1982.

In January of 1984, he gave up his engineering career to devote more time to research, writing, and teaching. In March of 1986, he purchased property in the Jamaica Plain area of Boston to be used as the headquarters of the new organization, Yang's Martial Arts Association (YMAA). The organization expanded to become a division of Yang's Oriental Arts Association, Inc. (YOAA).

In 2008, Dr. Yang began the nonprofit YMAA California Retreat Center. This training facility in rural California is where selected students enroll in a five-year residency to learn Chinese martial arts.

Dr. Yang has been involved in traditional Chinese wushu since 1961, studying Shaolin White Crane (Bai He), Shaolin Long Fist (Changquan), and taijiquan under several different masters. He has taught for more than forty-six years: seven years in Taiwan, five years at Purdue University, two years in Houston, twenty-six years in Boston, and more than eight years at the YMAA California Retreat Center. He has taught seminars all around the world, sharing his knowledge of Chinese martial arts and qigong in Argentina, Austria, Barbados, Botswana, Belgium, Bermuda, Brazil, Canada, China, Chile, England, Egypt, France, Germany, Holland, Hungary, Iceland, Iran, Ireland, Italy, Latvia, Mexico, New Zealand, Poland, Portugal, Saudi Arabia, Spain, South Africa, Switzerland, and Venezuela.

Since 1986, YMAA has become an international organization, which currently includes more than fifty schools located in Argentina, Belgium, Canada, Chile, France, Hungary, Ireland, Italy, New Zealand, Poland, Portugal, South Africa, Sweden, the United Kingdom, Venezuela, and the United States.

Many of Dr. Yang's books and videos have been translated into many languages, including French, Italian, Spanish, Polish, Czech, Bulgarian, Russian, German, and Hungarian.

Books by Dr. Yang, Jwing-Ming

Analysis of Shaolin Chin Na, 2nd ed. YMAA Publication Center, 1987, 2004

Ancient Chinese Weapons: A Martial Artist's Guide, 2nd ed. YMAA Publication Center, 1985, 1999

Arthritis Relief: Chinese Qigong for Healing & Prevention, 2nd ed. YMAA Publication Center, 1991, 2005

Back Pain Relief: Chinese Qigong for Healing and Prevention, 2nd ed. YMAA Publication Center, 1997, 2004

Baguazhang: Theory and Applications, 2nd ed. YMAA Publication Center, 1994, 2008

Comprehensive Applications of Shaolin Chin Na: The Practical Defense of Chinese Seizing Arts. YMAA Publication Center, 1995

Essence of Shaolin White Crane: Martial Power and Qigong. YMAA Publication Center, 1996

How to Defend Yourself. YMAA Publication Center, 1992

Introduction to Ancient Chinese Weapons. Unique Publications, Inc., 1985

Meridian Qigong, YMAA Publication Center, 2016

*Northern Shaolin Sword 2*nd *ed. YMAA Publication Center, 1985, 2000*

Qigong for Health and Martial Arts, 2nd ed. YMAA Publication Center, 1995, 1998

Qigong Massage: Fundamental Techniques for Health and Relaxation, 2nd ed. YMAA Publication Center, 1992, 2005

Qigong Meditation: Embryonic Breathing. YMAA Publication Center, 2003

Qigong Meditation: Small Circulation, YMAA Publication Center, 2006

Qigong, the Secret of Youth: Da Mo's Muscle/Tendon Changing and Marrow/Brain Washing Qigong, 2nd ed. YMAA Publication Center, 1989, 2000

Root of Chinese qigong: Secrets of qigong Training, 2nd ed. YMAA Publication Center, 1989, 1997

Shaolin Chin Na. Unique Publications, Inc., 1980

Shaolin Long Fist Kung Fu. Unique Publications, Inc., 1981

Simple Qigong Exercises for Health: The Eight Pieces of Brocade, 3rd ed. YMAA Publication Center, 1988, 1997, 2013

Tai Chi Ball Qigong: For Health and Martial Arts. YMAA Publication Center, 2010

Tai Chi Chuan Classical Yang Style: The Complete Long Form and Qigong, 2nd ed. YMAA Publication Center, 1999, 2010

Tai Chi Chuan Martial Applications, 2nd ed. YMAA Publication Center, 1986, 1996

Tai Chi Chuan Martial Power, 3rd ed. YMAA Publication Center, 1986, 1996, 2015

Tai Chi Chuan: Classical Yang Style, 2nd ed. YMAA Publication Center, 1999, 2010

Tai Chi qigong: The Internal Foundation of Tai Chi Chuan, 2nd ed. rev. YMAA Publication Center, 1997, 1990, 2013

Tai Chi Secrets of the Ancient Masters: Selected Readings with Commentary. YMAA Publication Center, 1999

Tai Chi Secrets of the Wŭ and Li Styles: Chinese Classics, Translation, Commentary. YMAA Publication Center, 2001

Tai Chi Secrets of the Wu Style: Chinese Classics, Translation, Commentary. YMAA Publication Center, 2002

Tai Chi Secrets of the Yang Style: Chinese Classics, Translation, Commentary. YMAA Publication Center, 2001

Tai Chi Sword Classical Yang Style: The Complete Long Form, qigong, and Applications, 2nd ed. YMAA Publication Center, 1999, 2014

Taiji Chin Na: The Seizing Art of Taijiquan, 2nd ed. YMAA Publication Center, 1995, 2014

Taijiquan Theory of Dr. Yang, Jwing-Ming: The Root of Taijiquan. YMAA Publication Center, 2003

Xingyiquan: Theory and Applications, 2nd ed. YMAA Publication Center, 1990, 2003

Yang Style Tai Chi Chuan. Unique Publications, Inc., 1981

Videos alphabetical

Advanced Practical Chin Na in Depth, YMAA Publication Center, 2010

Analysis of Shaolin Chin Na. YMAA Publication Center, 2004

Baguazhang (Eight Trigrams Palm Kung Fu). YMAA Publication Center, 2005

Chin Na in Depth: Courses 1–4. YMAA Publication Center, 2003

Chin Na in Depth: Courses 5–8. YMAA Publication Center, 2003

Chin Na in Depth: Courses 9–12. YMAA Publication Center, 2003

Five Animal Sports Qigong. YMAA Publication Center, 2008

Knife Defense: Traditional Techniques. YMAA Publication Center, 2011

Meridian Qigong, YMAA Publication Center, 2015

Neigong, YMAA Publication Center, 2015

Northern Shaolin Sword. YMAA Publication Center, 2009

Qigong Massage. YMAA Publication Center, 2005

Saber Fundamental Training. YMAA Publication Center, 2008

Shaolin Kung Fu Fundamental Training. YMAA Publication Center, 2004

Shaolin Long Fist Kung Fu: Basic Sequences. YMAA Publication Center, 2005

Shaolin Saber Basic Sequences. YMAA Publication Center, 2007

Shaolin Staff Basic Sequences. YMAA Publication Center, 2007

Shaolin White Crane Gong Fu Basic Training: Courses 1 & 2. YMAA Publication Center, 2003

Shaolin White Crane Gong Fu Basic Training: Courses 3 & 4. YMAA Publication Center, 2008

Shaolin White Crane Hard and Soft Qigong. YMAA Publication Center, 2003

Shuai Jiao: Kung Fu Wrestling. YMAA Publication Center, 2010

Simple Qigong Exercises for Arthritis Relief. YMAA Publication Center, 2007

Simple Qigong Exercises for Back Pain Relief. YMAA Publication Center, 2007

Simple Qigong Exercises for Health: The Eight Pieces of Brocade. YMAA Publication Center, 2003

Staff Fundamental Training: Solo Drills and Matching Practice. YMAA Publication Center, 2007

Sword Fundamental Training. YMAA Publication Center, 2009

Tai Chi Ball Qigong: Courses 1 & 2. YMAA Publication Center, 2006

Tai Chi Ball Qigong: Courses 3 & 4. YMAA Publication Center, 2007

Tai Chi Chuan: Classical Yang Style. YMAA Publication Center, 2003

Tai Chi Fighting Set: 2-Person Matching Set. YMAA Publication Center, 2006

Tai Chi Pushing Hands: Courses 1 & 2. YMAA Publication Center, 2005

Tai Chi Pushing Hands: Courses 3 & 4. YMAA Publication Center, 2006

Tai Chi Qigong. YMAA Publication Center, 2005

Tai Chi Sword, Classical Yang Style. YMAA Publication Center, 2005

Tai Chi Symbol: Yin/Yang Sticking Hands. YMAA Publication Center, 2008

Taiji 37 Postures Martial Applications. YMAA Publication Center, 2008

Taiji Chin Na in Depth. YMAA Publication Center, 2009

Taiji Saber: Classical Yang Style. YMAA Publication Center, 2008

Taiji Wrestling: Advanced Takedown Techniques. YMAA Publication Center, 2008

Understanding Qigong, DVD 1: What is Qigong? The Human Qi Circulatory System. YMAA Publication Center, 2006

Understanding Qigong, DVD 2: Key Points of Qigong & Qigong Breathing. YMAA Publication Center, 2006

Understanding Qigong, DVD 3: Embryonic Breathing. YMAA Publication Center, 2007

Understanding Qigong, DVD 4: Four Seasons Qigong. YMAA Publication Center, 2007

Understanding Qigong, DVD 5: Small Circulation. YMAA Publication Center, 2007

Understanding Qigong, DVD 6: Martial Arts Qigong Breathing. YMAA Publication Center, 2007

Xingyiquan: Twelve Animals Kung Fu and Applications. YMAA Publication Center, 2008

Yang Tai Chi for Beginners. YMAA Publication Center, 2012

YMAA 25-Year Anniversary. YMAA Publication Center, 2009

BOOKS FROM YMAA

101 REFLECTIONS ON TAI CHI CHUAN
108 INSIGHTS INTO TAI CHI CHUAN
A SUDDEN DAWN: THE EPIC JOURNEY OF BODHIDHARMA
A WOMAN'S QIGONG GUIDE
ADVANCING IN TAE KWON DO
ANALYSIS OF SHAOLIN CHIN NA 2ND ED
ANCIENT CHINESE WEAPONS
ART AND SCIENCE OF STAFF FIGHTING
ART AND SCIENCE OF STICK FIGHTING
ART OF HOJO UNDO
ARTHRITIS RELIEF, 3D ED.
BACK PAIN RELIEF, 2ND ED.
BAGUAZHANG, 2ND ED.
BRAIN FITNESS
CARDIO KICKBOXING ELITE
CHIN NA IN GROUND FIGHTING
CHINESE FAST WRESTLING
CHINESE FITNESS
CHINESE TUI NA MASSAGE
CHOJUN
COMPLETE MARTIAL ARTIST
COMPREHENSIVE APPLICATIONS OF SHAOLIN CHIN NA
CONFLICT COMMUNICATION
CUTTING SEASON: A XENON PEARL MARTIAL ARTS THRILLER
DAO DE JING
DAO IN ACTION
DEFENSIVE TACTICS
DESHI: A CONNOR BURKE MARTIAL ARTS THRILLER
DIRTY GROUND
DR. WU'S HEAD MASSAGE
DUKKHA HUNGRY GHOSTS
DUKKHA REVERB
DUKKHA, THE SUFFERING: AN EYE FOR AN EYE
DUKKHA UNLOADED
ENZAN: THE FAR MOUNTAIN, A CONNOR BURKE MARTIAL ARTS
    THRILLER
ESSENCE OF SHAOLIN WHITE CRANE
EVEN IF IT KILLS ME
EXPLORING TAI CHI
FACING VIOLENCE
FIGHT BACK
FIGHT LIKE A PHYSICIST
THE FIGHTER'S BODY
FIGHTER'S FACT BOOK
FIGHTER'S FACT BOOK 2
FIGHTING ARTS
FIGHTING THE PAIN RESISTANT ATTACKER
FIRST DEFENSE
FORCE DECISIONS: A CITIZENS GUIDE
FOX BORROWS THE TIGER'S AWE
INSIDE TAI CHI
JUDO ADVANTAGE
JUJI GATAME ENCYCLOPEDIA
KAGE: THE SHADOW, A CONNOR BURKE MARTIAL ARTS THRILLER
KARATE SCIENCE
KATA AND THE TRANSMISSION OF KNOWLEDGE
KRAV MAGA COMBATIVES
KRAV MAGA PROFESSIONAL TACTICS
KRAV MAGA WEAPON DEFENSES
LITTLE BLACK BOOK OF VIOLENCE
LIUHEBAFA FIVE CHARACTER SECRETS
MARTIAL ARTS ATHLETE
MARTIAL ARTS OF VIETNAM
MARTIAL ARTS INSTRUCTION
MARTIAL WAY AND ITS VIRTUES
MASK OF THE KING
MEDITATIONS ON VIOLENCE
MERIDIAN QIGONG EXERCISES
MIND/BODY FITNESS
MINDFUL EXERCISE
MIND INSIDE TAI CHI
MIND INSIDE YANG STYLE TAI CHI CHUAN
NATURAL HEALING WITH QIGONG
NORTHERN SHAOLIN SWORD, 2ND ED.
OKINAWA'S COMPLETE KARATE SYSTEM: ISSHIN RYU
PAIN-FREE BACK

PAIN-FREE JOINTS
POWER BODY
PRINCIPLES OF TRADITIONAL CHINESE MEDICINE
PROTECTOR ETHIC
QIGONG FOR HEALTH & MARTIAL ARTS 2ND ED.
QIGONG FOR LIVING
QIGONG FOR TREATING COMMON AILMENTS
QIGONG MASSAGE
QIGONG MEDITATION: EMBRYONIC BREATHING
QIGONG MEDITATION: SMALL CIRCULATION
QIGONG, THE SECRET OF YOUTH: DA MO'S CLASSICS
QUIET TEACHER: A XENON PEARL MARTIAL ARTS THRILLER
RAVEN'S WARRIOR
REDEMPTION
ROOT OF CHINESE QIGONG, 2ND ED.
SAMBO ENCYCLOPEDIA
SCALING FORCE
SELF-DEFENSE FOR WOMEN
SENSEI: A CONNOR BURKE MARTIAL ARTS THRILLER
SHIHAN TE: THE BUNKAI OF KATA
SHIN GI TAI: KARATE TRAINING FOR BODY, MIND, AND SPIRIT
SIMPLE CHINESE MEDICINE
SIMPLE QIGONG EXERCISES FOR HEALTH, 3RD ED.
SIMPLIFIED TAI CHI CHUAN, 2ND ED.
SOLO TRAINING
SOLO TRAINING 2
SPOTTING DANGER BEFORE IT SPOTS YOU
SUMO FOR MIXED MARTIAL ARTS
SUNRISE TAI CHI
SURVIVING ARMED ASSAULTS
TAE KWON DO: THE KOREAN MARTIAL ART
TAEKWONDO BLACK BELT POOMSAE
TAEKWONDO: A PATH TO EXCELLENCE
TAEKWONDO: ANCIENT WISDOM FOR THE MODERN WARRIOR
TAEKWONDO: DEFENSE AGAINST WEAPONS
TAEKWONDO: SPIRIT AND PRACTICE
TAI CHI BALL QIGONG: FOR HEALTH AND MARTIAL ARTS
TAI CHI BALL WORKOUT FOR BEGINNERS
THE TAI CHI BOOK
TAI CHI CHIN NA: THE SEIZING ART OF TAI CHI CHUAN,
    2ND ED.
TAI CHI CHUAN CLASSICAL YANG STYLE, 2ND ED.
TAI CHI CHUAN MARTIAL POWER, 3RD ED.
TAI CHI CONNECTIONS
TAI CHI DYNAMICS
TAI CHI FOR DEPRESSION
TAI CHI IN 10 WEEKS
TAI CHI PUSH HANDS
TAI CHI QIGONG, 3RD ED.
TAI CHI SECRETS OF THE ANCIENT MASTERS
TAI CHI SECRETS OF THE WU & LI STYLES
TAI CHI SECRETS OF THE WU STYLE
TAI CHI SECRETS OF THE YANG STYLE
TAI CHI SWORD: CLASSICAL YANG STYLE, 2ND ED.
TAI CHI SWORD FOR BEGINNERS
TAI CHI WALKING
TAIJIQUAN THEORY OF DR. YANG, JWING-MING
TAO OF BIOENERGETICS
TENGU: THE MOUNTAIN GOBLIN, A CONNOR BURKE MARTIAL ARTS
    THRILLER
TIMING IN THE FIGHTING ARTS
TRADITIONAL CHINESE HEALTH SECRETS
TRADITIONAL TAEKWONDO
TRAINING FOR SUDDEN VIOLENCE
TRUE WELLNESS
TRUE WELLNESS: THE MIND
TRUE WELLNESS FOR YOUR GUT
TRUE WELLNESS FOR YOUR HEART
WARRIOR'S MANIFESTO
WAY OF KATA
WAY OF SANCHIN KATA
WAY TO BLACK BELT
WESTERN HERBS FOR MARTIAL ARTISTS
WILD GOOSE QIGONG
WINNING FIGHTS
WISDOM'S WAY
XINGYIQUAN

DVDS FROM YMAA

ADVANCED PRACTICAL CHIN NA IN-DEPTH
ANALYSIS OF SHAOLIN CHIN NA
ATTACK THE ATTACK
BAGUA FOR BEGINNERS 1
BAGUA FOR BEGINNERS 2
BAGUAZHANG: EMEI BAGUAZHANG
BEGINNER QIGONG FOR WOMEN 1
BEGINNER QIGONG FOR WOMEN 2
BEGINNER TAI CHI FOR HEALTH
CHEN STYLE TAIJIQUAN
CHEN TAI CHI CANNON FIST
CHEN TAI CHI FIRST FORM
CHEN TAI CHI FOR BEGINNERS
CHIN NA IN-DEPTH COURSES 1—4
CHIN NA IN-DEPTH COURSES 5—8
CHIN NA IN-DEPTH COURSES 9—12
FACING VIOLENCE: 7 THINGS A MARTIAL ARTIST MUST KNOW
FIVE ANIMAL SPORTS
FIVE ELEMENTS ENERGY BALANCE
INFIGHTING
INTRODUCTION TO QI GONG FOR BEGINNERS
JOINT LOCKS
KNIFE DEFENSE: TRADITIONAL TECHNIQUES AGAINST A DAGGER
KUNG FU BODY CONDITIONING 1
KUNG FU BODY CONDITIONING 2
KUNG FU FOR KIDS
KUNG FU FOR TEENS
LOGIC OF VIOLENCE
MERIDIAN QIGONG
NEIGONG FOR MARTIAL ARTS
NORTHERN SHAOLIN SWORD : SAN CAI JIAN, KUN WU JIAN, QI MEN JIAN
QI GONG 30-DAY CHALLENGE
QI GONG FOR ANXIETY
QIGONG FOR BEGINNERS: FRAGRANCE
QI GONG FOR BETTER BALANCE
QI GONG FOR BETTER BREATHING
QI GONG FOR CANCER
QI GONG FOR DEPRESSION
QI GONG FOR ENERGY AND VITALITY
QI GONG FOR HEADACHES
QI GONG FOR HEALING
QI GONG FOR THE HEALTHY HEART
QI GONG FOR HEALTHY JOINTS
QI GONG FOR HIGH BLOOD PRESSURE
QIGONG FOR LONGEVITY
QI GONG FOR STRONG BONES
QI GONG FOR THE UPPER BACK AND NECK
QIGONG FOR WOMEN
QIGONG FOR WOMEN WITH DAISY LEE
QIGONG FLOW FOR STRESS & ANXIETY RELIEF
QIGONG MASSAGE
QIGONG MINDFULNESS IN MOTION
QI GONG—THE SEATED WORKOUT
QIGONG: 15 MINUTES TO HEALTH
SABER FUNDAMENTAL TRAINING
SAI TRAINING AND SEQUENCES
SANCHIN KATA: TRADITIONAL TRAINING FOR KARATE POWER
SCALING FORCE
SHAOLIN KUNG FU FUNDAMENTAL TRAINING: COURSES 1 & 2
SHAOLIN LONG FIST KUNG FU: ADVANCED SEQUENCES 1
SHAOLIN LONG FIST KUNG FU: ADVANCED SEQUENCES 2
SHAOLIN LONG FIST KUNG FU: BASIC SEQUENCES
SHAOLIN LONG FIST KUNG FU: INTERMEDIATE SEQUENCES
SHAOLIN SABER: BASIC SEQUENCES
SHAOLIN STAFF: BASIC SEQUENCES

SHAOLIN WHITE CRANE GONG FU BASIC TRAINING: COURSES 1 & 2
SHAOLIN WHITE CRANE GONG FU BASIC TRAINING: COURSES 3 & 4
SHUAI JIAO: KUNG FU WRESTLING
SIMPLE QIGONG EXERCISES FOR HEALTH
SIMPLE QIGONG EXERCISES FOR ARTHRITIS RELIEF
SIMPLE QIGONG EXERCISES FOR BACK PAIN RELIEF
SIMPLIFIED TAI CHI CHUAN: 24 & 48 POSTURES
SIMPLIFIED TAI CHI FOR BEGINNERS 48
SIX HEALING SOUNDS
SUNRISE TAI CHI
SUNSET TAI CHI
SWORD: FUNDAMENTAL TRAINING
TAEKWONDO KORYO POOMSAE
TAI CHI BALL QIGONG: COURSES 1 & 2
TAI CHI BALL QIGONG: COURSES 3 & 4
TAI CHI BALL WORKOUT FOR BEGINNERS
TAI CHI CHUAN CLASSICAL YANG STYLE
TAI CHI CONNECTIONS
TAI CHI ENERGY PATTERNS
TAI CHI FIGHTING SET
TAI CHI FIT: 24 FORM
TAI CHI FIT: FLOW
TAI CHI FIT: FUSION BAMBOO
TAI CHI FIT: FUSION FIRE
TAI CHI FIT: FUSION IRON
TAI CHI FIT: HEART HEALTH WORKOUT
TAI CHI FIT IN PARADISE
TAI CHI FIT: OVER 50
TAI CHI FIT OVER 50: BALANCE EXERCISES
TAI CHI FIT OVER 50: SEATED WORKOUT
TAI CHI FIT OVER 60: GENTLE EXERCISES
TAI CHI FIT OVER 60: HEALTHY JOINTS
TAI CHI FIT OVER 60: LIVE LONGER
TAI CHI FIT: STRENGTH
TAI CHI FIT: TO GO
TAI CHI FOR WOMEN
TAI CHI FUSION: FIRE
TAI CHI QIGONG
TAI CHI PUSHING HANDS: COURSES 1 & 2
TAI CHI PUSHING HANDS: COURSES 3 & 4
TAI CHI SWORD: CLASSICAL YANG STYLE
TAI CHI SWORD FOR BEGINNERS
TAI CHI SYMBOL: YIN YANG STICKING HANDS
TAIJI & SHAOLIN STAFF: FUNDAMENTAL TRAINING
TAIJI CHIN NA IN-DEPTH
TAIJI 37 POSTURES MARTIAL APPLICATIONS
TAIJI SABER CLASSICAL YANG STYLE
TAIJI WRESTLING
TRAINING FOR SUDDEN VIOLENCE
UNDERSTANDING QIGONG 1: WHAT IS QI? • HUMAN QI
    CIRCULATORY SYSTEM
UNDERSTANDING QIGONG 2: KEY POINTS • QIGONG BREATHING
UNDERSTANDING QIGONG 3: EMBRYONIC BREATHING
UNDERSTANDING QIGONG 4: FOUR SEASONS QIGONG
UNDERSTANDING QIGONG 5: SMALL CIRCULATION
UNDERSTANDING QIGONG 6: MARTIAL QIGONG BREATHING
WATER STYLE FOR BEGINNERS
WHITE CRANE HARD & SOFT QIGONG
YANG TAI CHI FOR BEGINNERS
YOQI QIGONG FLOW FOR HAPPY LUNGS
WUDANG KUNG FU: FUNDAMENTAL TRAINING
WUDANG SWORD
WUDANG TAIJIQUAN
XINGYIQUAN
YANG TAI CHI FOR BEGINNERS

more products available from . . .
YMAA Publication Center, Inc. 楊氏東方文化出版中心
1-800-669-8892 • info@ymaa.com • www.ymaa.com